UP THE CREEK

TRUE STORIES OF CANOEISTS IN TROUBLE

DOUG McKOWN, EDITOR

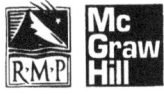

Ragged Mountain Press / McGraw-Hill
Camden, Maine • New York • Chicago • San Francisco • Lisbon
London • Madrid • Mexico City • Milan • New Delhi
San Juan • Seoul • Singapore • Sydney • Toronto

The McGraw-Hill Companies

1 2 3 4 5 6 7 8 9 1 0 DOC DOC 0 9 8 7 6 5 4

Library of Congress Cataloging-in-Publication Data
McKown, Doug, 1953–
  Up the creek : true stories of canoeists in trouble.
       p.   cm.
Includes bibliographical references.
  ISBN 0-07-139090-1
  1. Canoes and canoeing—Safety measures. 2. Canoeing accidents.
I. Title.
  GV784.55.M35 2004
  797.1′22′0289—dc22   2003022514

Questions regarding the content of this book should be addressed to
Ragged Mountain Press
P.O. Box 220
Camden, ME 04843
www.raggedmountainpress.com

Questions regarding the ordering of this book should be addressed to
The McGraw-Hill Companies
Customer Service Department
P.O. Box 547
Blacklick, OH 43004
Retail customers: 1-800-262-4729
Bookstores: 1-800-722-4726

Warning: Paddlesports can take paddlers into harm's way, exposing them
to risks of injury, cold-water exposure and hypothermia, drowning, and
other hazards that can lead to serious injury or death.
    This book is not intended to replace instruction by a qualified teacher
or to substitute for good personal judgment. In using this book, the reader
releases the author, publisher, and distributor from liability for any injury,
including death, that might result. It is understood that you paddle at your
own risk.

CONTENTS

INTRODUCTION

Y OBJECTIVE IN GATHERING these stories was to gain some idea of how and why canoeing accidents happen, in the hope that this information will help people paddle more safely. I soon realized that the term "accident" seems to be the justification of choice for anything bad that happens to a canoeist. "Accidents" are apparently all-inclusive, synonymous with "acts of God" and "random acts of nature." Skeptical, I delved into dictionaries in search of a more precise definition of an accident, and found my favorite: "an unfortunate event happening without intent, resulting from carelessness, unawareness, ignorance, or random, unpredictable factors." That covers just about everything! But how many "accidents" are actually preventable, I wondered, and how can paddlers best deal with the ones that are truly unavoidable? As I gathered more and more stories from experienced paddlers, I began to develop a much better appreciation of what really happens to canoeists when things go wrong.

These stories are all true accounts, related by the paddlers who experienced them. A couple of my sources wish to remain anonymous, and I have honored their requests ("A Tragedy on the Bow" and "Trouble on the Vermilion"). At the end of some stories, I've recapped the salient points in an editor's note.

In these stories, no surnames are given. Invented names first appear in quotation marks to indicate pseudonyms.

One of the terms used in the stories that might need clarification is "solo paddling," since there are two kinds of solo paddling. The first refers to one person paddling in a canoe. The second usually comes up in discussions of canoe safety, and there it refers to paddling with just one canoe, regardless of how many people are in it.

The problems that befall paddlers have many causes: poor planning, misjudgments, lack of skills, overconfidence, complacency, inattention, carelessness—the list goes on. It is hard to understand why skilled, experienced, reasonable, intelligent people make obvious misjudgments, disregard clear warning signs, ignore what experience tells them, and end up getting in trouble.

We expect problems and accidents from beginners, and indeed there are a few stories here which, though written by experienced paddlers, nevertheless recount how they survived early mistakes. These paddlers have come to realize just how unaware they were as novices. Beginners lack the knowledge and experience to understand what problems can develop, and therefore cannot be expected to judge the consequences of their actions, but this should not happen to experienced paddlers. As paddlers gain skill and experience, they should be better able to assess risks, make better judgments, and experience fewer problems. Or so you would think.

While history shows that people rarely learn from the mistakes of others, we *do* usually learn something from our *own* mistakes—provided we survive them. That makes it all the more interesting that the most experienced paddlers can do the silliest things. I know this from personal experience; I have more stories in here than anyone else. Faced with blindingly obvious facts and clear signals, paddlers will continue to ignore, underestimate, and misjudge them in the most blatant manner.

Hindsight is always 20/20. That is why stories like these can be useful. Collectively they illustrate what I feel to be the two primary building blocks of canoeing safety: pretrip planning and awareness.

These stories make clear what an amazing variety of things can go wrong on a canoe trip. But the point of the stories is not to expose and examine each little mistake, nor is it to teach you how to read a rapid or a map, use an ax, make a ferry glide, deal with an angry bear, recognize a changing weather pattern, or organize a group of paddlers. The goal, rather, is to bring to life the potentially serious, even deadly, consequences of just about every possible activity or decision on a canoe trip. I hope not to frighten you away from canoeing—far from it—but to help you recognize the critical importance of being as prepared as possible for any eventuality, and the importance of remaining constantly aware of the potential consequences of every action you take.

Hopefully these stories will help us all understand how easy it is to make a serious misjudgment, though that doesn't mean we will be able to prevent them all. Incidents are inevitable. The key to minimizing their consequences is early recognition and bringing the appropriate resources to bear—that is, safety awareness and preplanning. No matter how potentially disastrous an incident is, the severity of the consequences can usually be reduced with a timely intervention. Paddlers who maintain a constant awareness regarding their actions and their environment will be able to recognize when a bad decision is made or something is going wrong, and will intervene early with the necessary resources. Awareness is the key to safe canoeing. The earlier the recognition and the intervention, the better the outcome. When faced with a potentially disastrous situation, if every aspect of your intervention goes perfectly, you will experience no more than a close call, grist for campfire tales. You will have survived an incident that had the potential for disaster. Recognizing when you experience a close call may be the most important learning you can do.

CHAPTER ONE

LIVE AND LEARN—MAYBE

W E WERE ALL NOVICE PADDLERS ONCE, as the following stories make clear. In canoeing, whether you are a novice or an expert, the trouble with trouble is that it comes suddenly. In a flash, events are cascading out of control. You can only try to react to the situation—and hope to come out alive.

The key to avoiding trouble is anticipation, which is where beginning paddlers often go wrong. They simply lack the experience to see trouble over the horizon and deal with it. Trip leaders, for their part, sometimes err in not considering the skill levels of *all* trip participants.

The storytellers you're about to meet survived such missteps with a little luck. In retrospect, they recognize that these "interesting experiences" were in fact serious, even dangerous situations. Nietzsche's famous saying, "That which doesn't kill me makes me stronger," applies to paddling as well as to life. And if it doesn't make us stronger, at least it should make us a little smarter.

We paddlers—all of us—must continuously exercise our "safety awareness" muscles. By illustrating when and how fast trouble usually arrives, perhaps these stories will encourage everyone to greater preparation and vigilance.

LOST CANOE ON THE CLEARWATER RIVER
Dean Gyug

T HIS LITTLE ADVENTURE BEGAN in the middle of July, on the beautiful Clearwater River in northern Saskatchewan. It should have been a fine trip. We thought we were experienced. Janet and I were each paddling a solo river kayak, and Chris and Patrick had their open Grumman canoe. We had all paddled before, and a river canoe trip seemed like just the thing.

On day one we faced the big crossing of Lloyd Lake. The weather was foul and the wind was up, but we were able to organize a ride across the lake in a motorboat with friends from La Loche, Saskatchewan. We towed our kayaks and canoe across, arriving at the outlet of the Clearwater River after a wild two-hour ride. That first day on the river was pleasant, with a couple of good portages but no problems, and we began to feel pretty good.

Day two wasn't quite as happy. Our inexperience caught up with us a short distance upstream from a class 3+ rapid. Chris and Pat launched their canoe to paddle a little closer to the rapid, but somehow got into the heavily loaded canoe with only one paddle. Before they could get back to shore, they were swept into the powerful current. Unable to control their boat with one paddle, they carried on helplessly downstream, bouncing off rocks and taking on water. Things went rapidly from bad to worse as they headed toward the roaring rapids and Janet and I watched helplessly. Then the canoe, with Chris and Pat increasingly terrified, slammed broadside into a huge boulder.

Grumman aluminum canoes are notorious for sticking to rocks, and this one, true to form, was instantly stopped and pinned. The force of the impact ejected Chris from the front of the canoe, headfirst into the boulder-strewn river, where he hit his head hard. After a long and unpleasant swim, he eventually reached shore at the bottom of the rapid, bleeding from a nasty head wound. Meanwhile, Pat was thrown over the side of the canoe and into the eddy behind the boulder. He reached shore but had injured his leg. Most of the gear had disappeared down the rapid.

The four of us stood on the shore, looking at each other in disbelief. There we were, in the middle of northern Saskatchewan, with our Grumman canoe permanently, irretrievably wrapped around a midriver boulder and most of our gear lost. This wasn't good.

After portaging the two kayaks around the rapid, we sat down to take stock. Eventually Chris headed down the calm section of the river in one of the kayaks to try to retrieve some of our gear, while Janet, Pat, and I continued discussing how to extricate ourselves from the wilderness. The plan we settled on was that Chris and I would take the two kayaks the next day, aiming to reach the end of the river as soon as possible. Pat and Janet would remain at the camp. After two hours of effort, Chris managed to recover a paddle, a tent, two dry bags filled with equipment, and three sleeping bags.

The next morning Chris and I paddled off downriver. The road where we had planned to end the trip was 102 kilometers ahead. We took a fishing rod, two sleeping bags, and matches. Pat and Janet were left with the tent, rifle, cook set, dry food, and a few other odds and ends. They could be there as long as a week if things didn't go well for Chris and me.

Two long days of hard but very careful paddling carried us to the bridge. On such a remote road, however, this didn't mean immediate rescue. Another three days passed before a truck finally came by. The driver radioed for help, and three hours later a Royal Canadian Mounted Police officer arrived and drove us to La Loch. Only the next day were we able to organize a float-plane and head off to rescue Pat and Janet. They had been waiting five days. We were able to land on a small lake close to the river, and made a two-hour hike through dense bush to get to the campsite. To our great relief, Pat and Janet were fine, and *very* happy to see us.

We were lucky to come out of this trip as unscathed as we did. Chris suffered a concussion and Pat bruised legs and a sprained ankle, and we all gained a lot more respect for rivers. The experience instilled in all of us determination to develop the skills, training, and experience to safely enjoy an outing like this in the future. We completed the same trip two years later. Approaching the scene of our previous disaster, we saw the remains of our poor Grumman canoe, still pinned against that huge boulder.

EDITOR: *Proper pretrip planning and vital safety awareness come with experience, yet without planning and awareness it is impossible to assess your environment realistically and evaluate your actions appropriately. Therein lies the dilemma: how to acquire the experience without exposing oneself to danger in the process. In one guise or another, answering that question is the purpose of every story in this book.*

EXPERIENCE ON THE SLATER RIVER
Pam Little

I REALLY DON'T KNOW HOW I survived my first experience on moving water. Ignorance is bliss, I guess.

I had just graduated from university with a physical education degree and was a real jock. With a friend, Dianna, I visited my sister's place in southern Manitoba. Backing her farm is the Slater River, which flows into Duck Bay on Lake Winnipegosis. The Slater is a small river, but the spring melt had swollen it to full flood. My sister and brother-in-law were away, but my younger brother was there. We spent the morning stripping logs to build a cabin, until Dianna decided to take a break and had the brilliant idea that we should go for a paddle in my sister's Grumman aluminum canoe. We put the canoe into the river with me paddling stern, because I had done some lake canoeing as a summer camp counselor in the past, making me by far the more experienced paddler. The river roared along in a big brown flood. As soon as we launched we were swept downstream.

The river was so high it was overflowing its banks, and bushes and trees hung over the water. Willows slapped our faces, and we had absolutely no control of the canoe. After a while we came to appreciate those willows, and kept grabbing them to slow our stampede in the fast-flowing current. We broached on rocks but managed to get the sticky aluminum canoe free before it could capsize. Cows grazing in bordering pastures watched with apparent amusement as we spun helplessly past.

We had told my younger brother we were just going to paddle to a road about fifteen minutes downriver, but when he drove there we were nowhere in sight. I barely saw that road when we went past it, we were traveling so fast and so out of control. I was sure we would wash out into Duck Bay, which was miles away, but before that could happen we came to a huge eddy at a cattle crossing. The river chose to wash us into the eddy, and we managed finally to grab some trees and bring ourselves to a stop. By this time my sister was home, and she was frantic. She understood how dangerous that river can be.

We crawled out of the river and made our way back to the house. That was my introduction to river canoeing, and having survived that through no effort of our own, I have been having fun on rivers ever since.

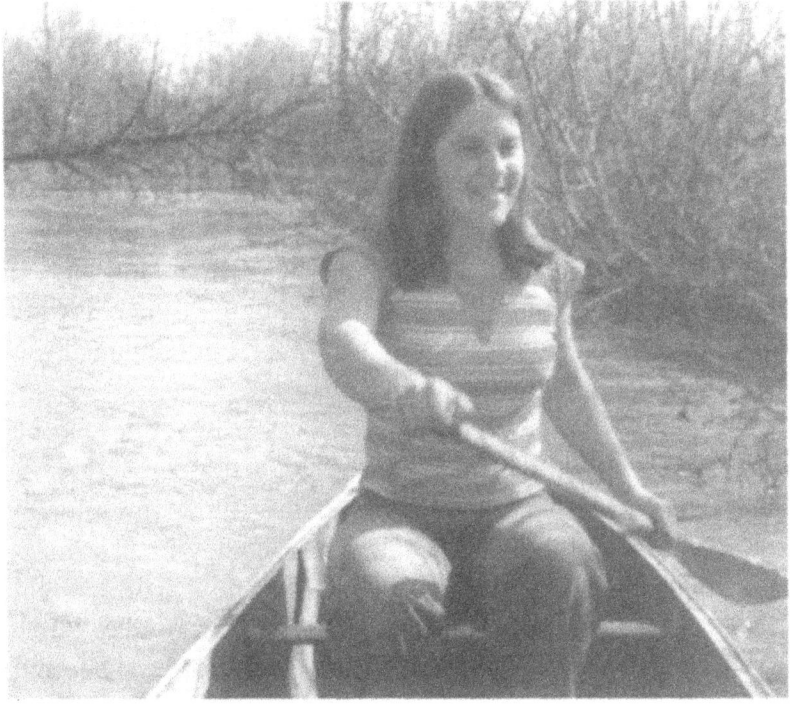

Pam Little about to head down the Slater River.

MY FIRST WILDERNESS RAPID—
AND ALMOST MY LAST

John Lentz

W HEN FRIENDS ASKED ME TO JOIN their four-person canoe expedition down the Back River in the Northwest Territories, I visited a local library to peruse Captain George Back's journal. His 1834 run with nine men in a longboat is an early classic of barrenlands travel. Struck by Back's vivid narration of some near "train wrecks" in the whitewater, I attempted to dissuade the others from going, but they convinced me we'd be fine.

Leaving Sussex Lake, the source of the Back, on July 13, we were full of confidence. Three of us had been counselors at boys' camps in Ontario and the fourth had recently been a member of the Harvard crew team. Our collective outdoor résumés had prepared us for lake paddling and minor riffles, but handling heavy water was a different matter.

The first few days were benign: class 1–2 rapids, easy current, and expanses of flatwater. But at noon on July 17 we saw the river fall away sharply to the right and heard the unmistakable roar of a serious rapid ahead. It was marked on our eight-miles-to-the-inch maps (all that was available at the time) with a double hash mark, still a few miles above the well-known Malley Rapid.

We eased our two eighteen-foot wood-and-canvas Chestnut Ogilvy canoes ashore at the top on river right to scout the hazard, and this was where we made our first mistake. We held a scouting discussion at the head of the rapid without taking the trouble to walk all or even part of its length. We decided we could run it by starting on river right, then moving most of the way across in the eddy of a huge rock, and finishing through a V-shaped chute on the left. But when this decision was made, we were at least eighty yards upstream of the final part of the route.

My partner, Tracy, and I shoved off first—kneeling on our life jackets. With near-perfect weather and having pronounced the rapid runnable, we just didn't feel threatened enough to put them on. We weren't even concerned enough to notice our long stern line trailing snakelike behind us. Everything went as planned until we reached the brink of that last chute, only to see a three-foot vertical drop into some nasty back curlers, a feature hidden from our distant scouting position. I sucked air and paddled hard from the bow in an attempt to punch through, but the loaded boat quickly began taking water in the standing waves.

The big canoe wallowed, then rolled. My first thought on bobbing to the surface was just to hold onto our faithful Chestnut and ride it out, but the trailing stern line had a knot in the end (someone's great idea) that became wedged in the rocks. The canoe was not only held fast but levered under, as if the river was eager to claim its due—a pair of pretty clueless paddlers. From my vantage point, floating away downstream, it was seriously intimidating to think that wood-and-canvas canoes didn't float on northern rivers!

Fortunately, my life jacket was close at hand, and I grabbed it and swam to one of the bobbing packs for more flotation. I still felt in control, with my feet downstream and head upstream, as I bounced through a small tailrace rapid. At the bottom, however, my head was pulled under, giving me a mouthful of forty-two-degree water and a dose of panic.

Tracy was a few meters off, astride a large camera box, shouting encouragement. Some minutes passed as we tried to kick for shore, but instead the bank receded. We were held in the grip of a powerful current that carried us toward a large lake expansion.

My first realization that this dump was far from routine came when my fingers began to straighten, losing their grip on the pack. There was no pain, just a scary realization that my brain could no longer command my hand. Before long I was clutching the pack with my forearm. Kicking became progressively more difficult. My body was protecting its core at the expense of its periphery as it reacted to the onset of hypothermia. Tracy was in better shape, since he had a larger frame and more of it was out of the frigid water.

After a few more minutes I became pretty much resigned to fate. Looking down, I could see small, colorful stones ten feet down as I swept past. "This just isn't right, I'm not supposed to be able to see my grave," was one morale-sapping thought. Then I tilted my head back and looked up at the gorgeous blue sky, thinking "What a lovely day to die." Tracy grabbed at me a few times, but was struggling to survive himself.

It was with some surprise that I felt Kit's (the Harvard crew man) strong hand on the back of my shirt, lifting me out of the drink and into his canoe. Fortunately, he and Austin had reacted as rescuers should—hurriedly wading down the edge of the rapid and emptying their boat before coming out to us (at least we hadn't committed both canoes to the rapid at the same time). My next sensation was being shoved into Kit's bedroll in my now lovingly familiar tent. Despite dry clothing, it took half an hour in the bedroll for me to stop shivering and for my breathing to calm down. Austin later told me that I was unable to unbutton my shirt when they deposited me on shore, but at least my speech was not slurred—a dangerous sign that even the brain has begun to feel the effects.

Tracy didn't require the bedroll treatment; leaping over rocks was enough to restore his circulation. While I recovered, the other

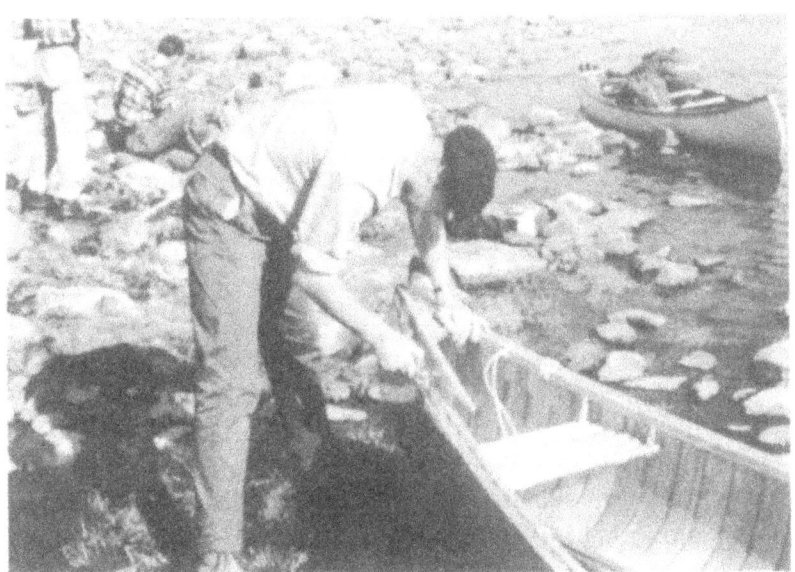

Making repairs after the capsize.

three cut our canoe loose from the boulders upstream and began to repair a split gunwale and a stern abrasion.

By midafternoon we had struck "camp" and were paddling down a lake expansion, although I still felt residual shivers. As Captain Back said when trying to inspire his men, "On to the Polar Sea!"

Those interminable minutes in the Back River a long time ago were as close as I've come to cashing in during my eighteen wilderness canoe trips. For the rest of the trip, we were as careful as possible. We had to be, or our trip might have ended at the next rapid. But in a broader sense, I came away with a new sense of conservatism when paddling remote rivers. I still take some chances, but only after making a complete appraisal of the situation, and with a bias toward the less risky option.

GOOD-BYE TO AN OLD FRIEND

Doug McKown

T HE WATER LEVEL IN THE VERMILION RIVER, in Kootenay National Park, British Columbia, was very high that day. Our party was made up of eight paddlers in four open canoes, along with myself in my C-1—a small, closed-deck, solo canoe. Seven of us were experienced river paddlers and had run this section of river before. The remaining two, Lynn and Karen, had flatwater experience but were new to rivers. We were on a section that was highly technical for the open canoes, with continuous rock gardens, ledges, and little canyons. I led the way in my C-1, and for a while things went well.

Eventually, however, we reached a canyon that was a little too pushy for the open canoes, so we decided to run them halfway down the canyon, one at a time, carry around the tricky bit, and finally line the canoes the rest of the way to the bottom. I paddled down in my C-1, parked just below the tricky bit, and walked back upstream along the bank to assist the other paddlers or use my throw bag if necessary. The first two canoes came down fine, and we carried them around the tough section. I got back into my C-1 when the third canoe arrived, since we now had ample people on shore. All three groups then started to line their canoes down the bank. As they headed away from me, walking along the edge of a two-meter cliff while lining the canoes on ropes, I realized our group was getting too spread out. I shouted upriver to the fourth canoe, asking them to wait, then turned back toward the lining operation. The river there was very narrow, smooth but fast.

Lynn and Karen, the second pair, were lining their Brigden Model 3 canoe. Lynn had hold of the downstream end rope of the canoe, Karen the upstream. Everything was simple and working as it should, but an instant later chaos ensued. The upstream end of the Brigden canoe swung out from shore into the current. Karen noticed it and pulled on her rope. Lynn felt the pressure on her rope and pulled on the downstream end as well. With tension on both ropes, the current caught the canoe and immediately flipped it upstream in the powerful current.

Once the canoe capsized, the force of the river on the hull was tremendous. Unable to withstand it, both women let go their ropes, luckily before either of them was pulled into the river. This whole sequence took about two seconds to unfold, and then we all watched as the canoe swirled away in the current.

I shouted, "Boat over!" and headed downstream after the canoe. With our last canoe still upstream, and no one else in a position to get into a canoe, I was on my own. While I had no problem looking after my C-1 on this river, I was completely unable to deal with a lone open canoe. I couldn't tie myself to it or try to T-rescue it. There was just too much maneuvering to be done. I kept nattering away at it, pushing and pulling, trying to get it hung up somewhere. I was forced to watch as, every time it went through rocks, it disintegrated a little more. First the thwarts went, then the seats, then the flotation chambers, then the hull started to break up.

After two or three kilometers I finally got it aimed at a gravel bar, where it ground to a halt in the shallows. There wasn't much left. The gunwales were gone, and while the hull was still in one piece, that piece had way more edges than it used to. When the rest of the group caught up to me, we collected the bits and dragged the whole mess up through the woods to the highway.

It's always sad to see a well-loved canoe destroyed. If it's going to happen, lining is one of the most likely ways. When novices are lining, their first impulse is to immediately pull back if they feel the current grab the boat—precisely the wrong thing to do. The situation could have been prevented if either Lynn or Karen had simply eased out her rope. If the downstream paddler, Lynn, had let go, the canoe would have swung parallel to the current and come harmlessly back to shore. If Karen had let go, the canoe would have swung around in the current and, again, come harmlessly back to shore.

If there is one cardinal rule in lining, it is simply, "when things go wrong, just let go."

CHAPTER TWO

THE RIGHT TOOL FOR THE RIGHT JOB

ROPERLY MAINTAINED, GOOD-QUALITY equipment rarely fails. Old or unfamiliar equipment can kill you, as can the loss of equipment. Experienced paddlers bring the right equipment and keep it in good shape. They know their lives may depend on it. Beginners often borrow equipment they aren't familiar with or bring insufficient or inappropriate equipment for the conditions they are likely to encounter.

Making sure equipment is up to the task is a matter of pretrip planning and organization. I prefer not to have anyone else organize my equipment and supplies. If you want to make sure everything is done right, do it yourself. A few days into a wilderness canoe trip is the wrong time to find out that you don't have what you need or that what you do have won't do the job.

Proper equipment should be one of the easiest elements of pretrip planning. But always remember that your equipment can be your best friend or your worst enemy.

SWAMPING ON THE SWAMPY BAY RIVER

Sara Seager and Mike Wevrick

THE SWAMPY BAY–CANIAPISCAU–KOKSOAK RIVER route in Québec is a marvelous canoe trip because the scenery changes constantly on the journey north from the Swampy Bay's headwaters near Schefferville to the mouth of the Koksoak at Ungava Bay. There are several breathtaking waterfalls and few, if any, other canoeists. Many sets of challenging rapids and rough portages make this a tough trip. The Swampy Bay follows a sheltered valley harboring a thicker cover of bushes and trees than at similar latitudes elsewhere, and deadfalls are frequent. There are almost no portage trails.

We spent a month on the river in the summer of 1999, taking a PakCanoe to avoid transportation hassles. This folding canoe handles quite unlike a rigid boat, mostly because it flexes going over waves.

Our trouble began about halfway through the trip, just after an incredibly tough portage. Thick bushes and deadfall lined the banks, and the only way around the rapid was up a steep hill and then back down. The deadfall looked like huge stacks of pickup sticks, often several logs deep. We had no choice but to climb over them. The PakCanoe was irritating to carry because it kept flexing and catching on brush. The portage made my back sore, even though the canoe weighed just fifty pounds (at least thirty pounds lighter than the Tripper I usually carry).

Although the next rapid was fairly long, I used my binoculars instead of scouting its entire length, something I usually wouldn't do. I did notice a line of white (a ledge), which should have set off alarm bells, as it was visible from a distance. The canoe was new, and we hadn't been able to test it before leaving because the shallow and rocky rivers near our home would have damaged it. Our cursory scouting complete, we started down.

The rapid was much pushier and more technical than we had expected, and it required all our concentration to maneuver the fully loaded boat. Mike was in the front, I was in back. We usually choose these positions for technical, low-volume rapids because Mike has quicker reflexes and better eyesight, but since he is heavier, we avoid this arrangement when running high-volume rapids. This rapid was fast, with a string of large boulders to maneuver through. Still, it offered nothing we hadn't done before.

Almost immediately, however, we went through a small hole, and a wave came over the bow. The weight of the water, coupled with Mike's weight, pulled down the front of the boat. With the next wave, we began to take on water. Due to the canoe's lack of rigidity, I couldn't see that the entire bow was swamping.

Mike looked back at me—something he never does in rapids—with an expression I have only seen twice before (including once when we were trapped in a forest fire and almost died), but I still didn't know what was wrong. Then he was in the water, and my end of the boat quickly filled too.

The rapid was studded with huge boulders (seven or eight feet high) separated by deep water. We were moving fast down the middle of the river, which at this point was about thirty to forty feet wide. We could only hold onto the back of the canoe in an attempt to guide it to the main shoreline without letting it broach—a disaster for such a fragile canoe. The salesperson had claimed it could be patched even if shredded from wrapping, but we didn't want to put that pronouncement to the test. Even resting against a boulder was a bad idea because of potential canoe damage.

Kira, our dog, was standing on top of a pack in the swamped canoe, not sure what to do. I grabbed her life jacket handle and lifted her onto a passing boulder. She started barking wildly, afraid we were abandoning her in the middle of a long, fierce rapid. What a place! I wonder what was going through her mind when she saw us moving quickly downstream and realized there was only one alternative—jump into the froth. Usually we leave Kira on shore when running tough rapids, and she meets us at the bottom. But just then she was the least of our worries. She knows how to swim in rapids, and her excellent life jacket provides additional flotation.

We finally got ourselves and the canoe to shore with no serious damage. Kira was right behind us. We stopped for a hot lunch and then portaged the rest of the rapid. After more climbing over deadfalls and breaking through a thicket of willows to reach the river again, we were exhausted. The long swim and the tension had worn us out, even though we weren't harmed by the mishap. It was an easy decision to camp right there.

Nothing inside the packs got wet, and we didn't lose anything, which was a good test of our packing strategy. We hadn't even tied anything into the canoe, since we had been afraid that floating packs would tear the vinyl boat to shreds. Luckily, the water and air were relatively warm (both around sixty degrees), and we were well dressed (I was wearing one layer of polypro, one of wool, and one of Gore-Tex).

What did we do wrong? We failed to scout well because we were feeling lazy after dealing with the deadfalls and brush on the previous portage. And we had become complacent about rapids, ignoring telltale signs (such as a ledge and big waves) because we'd tackled similar rapids many times before, though with a different canoe. Most importantly, we had failed to test our new boat before using it in a potentially dangerous situation.

The event had a serious effect on me during the rest of the trip. I acquired a strong aversion to paddling anything more than class 1 rapids, especially on cold, rainy mornings, and only pad-dled those in search of a portage just before a falls. Finally, just before our fifth portage of a dark, overcast day about four days later, Mike had had enough carrying. He said he was going to paddle the canoe, and that if I wasn't going to join him I would have to carry the packs myself, since he couldn't solo with the canoe fully loaded. I didn't want to paddle the rapids, but, the portage option seemed worse—totally dense brush with lots of deadfall. I paddled.

As soon as we were in the big waves I began to enjoy myself—it was a blast! This time there were no rocks. I like to think that first swamping on a northern river will keep me from ever be-coming complacent again, but only time will tell.

A CLOSE CALL

George Drought

W E HELD A FINAL MEETING in a motel room in Hearst, in northern Ontario. The meeting was critical because the next day we would be on an Algoma Central train traveling south to the whistle-stop village of Oba, where we would catch a train east to Peterbell, on the Missinaibi River. This was our chance to check that every member of the party had what they needed for the expedition. My wife, Barbara, and I already prepared the food and canoes, but we still had to issue tents, paddles, and PFDs before shuttling the trailer back to the take-out at Mattice.

After discussing logistics, we all went out to the trailer and unloaded the canoes and food, and paddlers off-loaded tents, paddles, and PFDs as needed. That evening we enjoyed a delicious dinner at the motel.

Early the next morning, I was loading canoes and equipment onto a freight car when Harry walked up and asked, "George, do you have my PFD?"

"No!" I replied. "You should have gotten it out of the trailer last night as we arranged at the meeting."

"Oh, I misunderstood you," he responded.

The train was leaving in ten minutes. The PFD Harry needed was in the trailer twenty kilometers away, and due to the early hour, all the stores in Hearst were closed. I asked one of the railmen if there were any PFDs available around the station, but nothing turned up. There was nothing to do but load ourselves on the train.

Barbara, Harry, and I discussed the options: I could lend Harry my PFD to run rapids, and then he or I would have to walk the portage to recover the PFD so that the other could enjoy the run; or, I could inflate a Therm-a-Rest and wrap it securely around myself as a makeshift PFD. Neither solution was really satisfactory.

While we were throwing out ideas, the conductor walked through checking tickets. Knowing that Oba was a very small town, I asked him if there was anyone on the train or in Oba who might sell us a PFD. He went off to check with the engineer, and half an hour later returned to say that someone named George in Oba might be able to help. He gave me directions to George's house and wished us luck. We needed it. The thought of spending ten days on the Missinaibi short one PFD was not appealing.

Fortunately, we had four hours to kill in Oba before the eastbound train was due. I wasted no time in following the conductor's directions and soon was traveling down a narrow trail among high willows. It opened into a clearing that contained a small dwelling covered with tar paper. I knocked on the door and heard some scuffling before a man's lean, unshaven face appeared to ask what I wanted. After I explained my situation, his response was to ask me how many were in our group and then to tell me to return to the station. He would see what he could do and would be there in about half an hour. I left, still none the wiser about whether we had found a PFD.

Right on time, George arrived at the station wearing green work clothes and carrying a large, steaming kettle in one hand and a green garbage bag in the other. "Would you like some wild mint tea?" he asked the assembled and expectant canoeists. "And oh, yes! I have a life jacket. Just bought it a week ago for $35 and it's yours for the same." Out of the garbage bag, he pulled the PFD, a new Buoy-o-Buoy. It fit Harry perfectly.

EDITOR: *Not a very exciting story? Well, that's the whole point. The importance of proper equipment in the wilderness cannot be overemphasized, which is why George went to such trouble to secure that missing life jacket.*

BIG WAVES AND SMALL CANOES
Jim Buckingham

VERY FRIDAY NIGHT FROM early May to late September used to find us down at the Winnipeg Canoe Club loading boats for a weekend trip to the lake country of eastern Manitoba and western Ontario. That region is great for short canoe trips, as there are countless small lakes connected by short portages.

One year someone decided we should end the paddling season by having Thanksgiving dinner on a canoe trip. We would paddle and portage to a remote lake, set up camp on Saturday, spend most of Sunday preparing and eating a multicourse turkey dinner, and then paddle back to the roadhead on the holiday Monday (Thanksgiving is celebrated on the second Monday in October in Canada). In Manitoba, the weather in October ranges from beautiful, warm Indian summer days and cool evenings to "snowin' and blowin'," so we knew we were pushing it.

As luck would have it, this particular Thanksgiving weekend was cold. By the time we finished the last portage into our destination lake, the wind was blowing pretty hard and a serious chop had kicked up. It soon became obvious that we would be foolish to try for the campsite at the far end of the lake, which involved crossing an open expanse with no shelter from the wind. Instead, we set up camp on a heavily wooded point. We were safely out of the wind there, and Sunday's Thanksgiving dinner was great.

Monday morning, however, we had to face the music. It was

snowing, with a strong, cold wind out of the north. For the first mile the wind would be hard on our backs, and the waves would be high. It wasn't a good day for swimming.

Our mixed flotilla started down the lake chased by big waves and the cold wind. Most of us were in the club's Brigden Model 20 sixteen-foot canoes—long, very narrow, distinctly V-shaped hulls that conformed to the length restrictions for the long-distance races our club members sometimes entered. These canoes were light, fast, and in fact were excellent for weekend canoe trips on sheltered lakes. With light camping gear, a couple could make single-trip portages and just fly through the lakes, seeing a lot of country on a weekend. The club also owned a couple of wider canoes, Brigden Model 3s with lines more like Chestnut Prospectors or Grummans. These were much better boats in waves and with big loads, but if you took one on a trip where everyone else was paddling the fast boats, all you saw of anyone else was their backsides, and even then you only saw them from a long way back. Anticipating rough water, a few of our party were in Model 3s.

There was yet another canoe with us, too—the club's twenty-five-foot war canoe, which was quite comfortable in big waves. For an easy weekend trip with less experienced paddlers, we used to pile the rookies into this big canoe with a couple of veterans and head out. Portages were a bit tough, but manageable with lots of bodies. That canoe was deep and could carry an enormous load.

Soon the experienced paddlers in the fast little boats were getting a great ride. If you sat the waves just right you could surf on every wave. For one of the Model 20s, though, it was a little more difficult. This canoe contained the chief cook and organizer of the dinner and was packed with cooking equipment and leftover food. He was a good paddler, but neither he nor the woman he was paddling with was small. Their canoe was sitting an inch or two deeper in the water than everyone else's, and this proved to be critical.

When we hit the middle of the most open stretch we had to cross, his canoe started taking waves over the stern. Each little wave left the canoe a little deeper in the water. There was nothing he could do, and the result was inevitable. Eventually the gunwales sank below the surface, and they were swamped. And there they were, a good couple hundred yards from shore, desperately clinging to a swamped canoe while cold waves broke over their heads and a wind-driven snow blanketed the waters.

Fortunately the group had stayed close together, and the war canoe was right there. Properly controlled, it was perfectly comfortable in the big waves and blowing snow. Its crew couldn't get the two swimmers out of the water, but they did rescue all the floating gear and towed the swimmers quickly to shore, hypothermic (though no one really understood hypothermia back then) but otherwise OK. We warmed them up with a fire and hot tea and chocolate bars, gave them dry clothes, and redistributed our loads. With the worst stretch behind us, we reached the portage without further incident.

The next lake was rough as well, so most of us decided not to risk it, opting instead to stay overnight near the portage. Some people felt obligated to be at work the next morning, so they waited until evening when the wind subsided and made it safely back to their cars in the dark. The rest of us set out early the next morning before the wind picked up. A few students missed some classes, and others had to do a lot of explaining to their bosses, but everyone got home safely—and there was considerable thanks-giving for that.

EDITOR: *The larger the group—and the greater the variety of equipment in use—the harder it is to recognize when a little problem is developing into a potentially deadly situation. Bringing the large war canoe along as a safety boat was part of the pretrip planning that kept this group safe in tough conditions.*

RANDOM ACTS OF NATURE

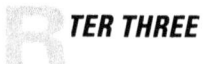**TER THREE**

ANDOM ACTS OF NATURE CAN COME in many forms: intense storms, unusually high water conditions, wild animals, forest fires, or any rapid, unexpected change in conditions. While these events are unpredictable, it is possible to plan for them and equip yourself accordingly. This is an integral part of proper planning and organization. The consequences of an act of nature often hinge on your preparation.

Your response to a situation is equally critical. Nature's random acts are rarely instantaneous, and safety awareness is your best defense. Pay close attention to weather changes, deteriorating hydraulic conditions, signs of wildlife, and the condition of your group so you'll be able to make early, correct decisions to head off trouble. Hopefully, your preplanning will provide you with the resources and options to make a successful response. Don't remain far offshore as rough weather approaches or erect your tent beside a dead tree just because you expect calm conditions or assume a distant forest fire won't change direction.

Animals in particular provide many interesting encounters. Anyone who spends much time in the outdoors will probably have to deal with bears at some point. Still, I was surprised by the number of bear stories I received while compiling this book. It seems that every experienced wilderness paddler has at least one.

Don't be surprised when nature decides to test you. Think ahead, plan adequately, and stay alert. And if you are faced with a potentially dangerous situation, react with your head—don't panic.

WHITEWATER WITH A TWIST

Dave Christopherson

WE WERE HIDING FROM THE WIND among the islands at the entrance to Guncoat Bay, on the Churchill River in Saskatchewan, one July day. After making a chocolate layer cake to pass the time, Wayne, Jean, and I decided to explore the islands while James and David J., the two teenagers in our group, opted to laze about on the small island where we were camped.

Out among the islands, Jean made good time in the solo boat and Wayne and I were happy with the quick, responsive performance of the sixteen-foot Prospector we were paddling. This area of the Churchill River system demonstrates the classic beauty of the Canadian Shield—rocks, water, and trees arranged in a soul-pleasing pattern. The waves on the open water of the bay had dropped enough to tempt us to pack up and continue on toward Nistowiak Falls, but it was getting on in the day, and we were in no rush to fight the rough water. There is always another day, another trip.

It was near midafternoon, and we could see thunderclouds begin to build up to the south. Time to end our exploration and head back to camp. There was no need to stay out and test our rain gear when a dry tarp and warm fire awaited. We moved all three canoes to a better landing site than the one we had used the night before. Jean, true to form, ensured that the canoes were securely tied to a strong clump of willows.

We were enjoying a warm drink under the tarp when the

clouds rolled over. The faucet opened, engulfing us in the deluge. Heavy rain—or any storm—can be a lot of fun to watch from a protected viewpoint. And it was coming down hard. The water in front of us was still fairly calm but covered in a solid mat of tiny raindrop explosions—complemented by intermittent hail.

Suddenly the wind veered, blowing the downpour straight into our faces. As luck would have it, I was the only one wearing rain gear. While the others frantically dove for their tents, I stayed out among the trees to enjoy the show. As an old salt once said, "The wind she blow, and by-and-by she blow some more."

While I watched, the wind turned the tarp into a large horizontal sail. I thought about trying to wrestle it to the ground but decided instead to check on Jean and our tent, which was tucked into a small clearing in the middle of the island.

The wind really let loose just as I crawled into the tent, where Jean was still changing out of wet clothing. I had experienced strong winds before, but nothing like the force that was coming through the trees and pushing down on one side of our tent—collapsing the wall on me while I lay stretched out on my Therm-a-Rest. For perhaps two or three minutes I lay there stupefied by the wind, thinking, "Good grief, I feel like we're in a tornado!"

As quickly as they struck, the powerful winds disappeared, and we were in dead calm. We heard Wayne call out, "Stay in your tents. We are in the eye!" Unknown to me, Wayne and James had emerged from their tents at about the same time I had dived into mine.

During this dead calm, which may have lasted thirty seconds, Jean looked over and said, "Well, if I'm going to die I am damn well going to die with my pants on." She had no sooner started suiting up than the wind came smashing in from the opposite direction. Again the tent was pushed down on us. This time, moreover, I could hear trees falling. When the wind let up two or three minutes later, Jean asked why the tent wall was still pushed in. Had one of the poles been damaged by the wind? Not so. The top of a fifty-foot spruce tree had landed beside our tent, pressing in on one wall.

Outside, everything looked different. Trees were down everywhere. We couldn't take more than ten steps in any direction without crawling over one or several fallen trees. Thankfully, no one was hurt. Even more amazing, with the exception of the shredded tarp, no equipment was damaged or missing. The canoes that Jean had secured so carefully had been picked up, shuffled in order, and deposited neatly in a clump of willows with their tie-down ropes pulled taut. Without Jean's insistence on always tying them up, the canoes would have been long gone.

Wayne and James had been looking out at the lake when the tornado struck. Within a minute, the small chop that had been livening the lake surface was replaced by four-foot waves racing down the channel. The wind literally stripped the water off the waves and threw it up in the air, creating a fifty- or sixty-foot wall of mist so dense that Wayne and James couldn't see across the channel to a point less than two hundred meters away.

When the eye of the tornado passed over us, they could see a strangely yellow sky through the funnel. They also saw the next wall of wind ready to blast us from the opposite direction, dropping many of the already weakened trees. Fortunately, the fallen trees caught Wayne's tent as it was torn from the ground.

Throughout this ordeal, David J. was alone in the tent that he shared with James. Two trees had fallen on the tent, but he emerged unscathed. While he didn't say much about this, it was apparent that his adrenaline was pumping, because in short order there were paths cut through the maze of fallen trees and we were able to move easily around the transformed island.

After cleaning up and reorganizing our devastated campsite, we sat down to enjoy a warm drink while marveling about how lucky we were. We were just getting comfortable when James and I glanced at the sky. "Don't look now," he said, "but I think another tornado is starting to form." The clouds to the southwest had started to spin in a large circular pattern. For the next hour we sat watching in awe and fear as a huge inverted bell devel-

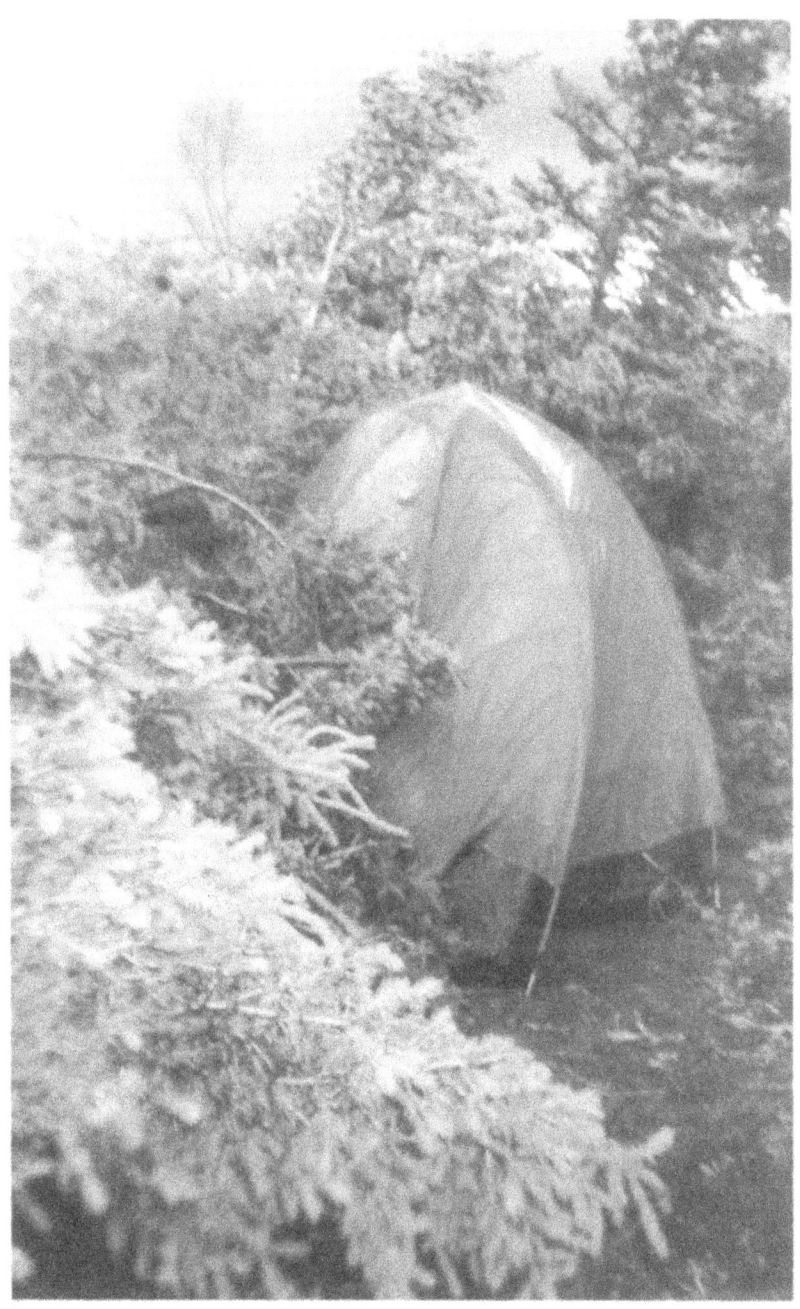

A close call when this tree just missed our tent.

oped, slowly reaching down until it touched ground. Hitting just beyond a point of land to the west of us, this large tornado continued north, spinning off at least six narrow, high-velocity funnel clouds as it moved. It slowly dissipated into one of the largest thunderclouds I've ever seen.

Living through a tornado and being right in the eye of the storm was incredibly frightening; however, watching that second tornado form up and touch down so close had to be the most terrifying experience of my life. We were totally at the mercy of the forces of nature, powerless to protect ourselves.

Even though we felt incredibly fortunate, we had no idea just how lucky we were. Two weeks later Jean and I were heading even farther north for a second canoe trip. As we were passing Missinipe, there was a break in what had been almost a week of continuous rain. On a whim, we decided to charter a floatplane to look at the landscape where the tornado had struck.

The small island where we had been camped looked beaten up but still forested. The larger islands just to the north and south looked as if a rotary mower had leveled them.

There was not a shred of green to be seen, and the trees, bare of leaves or needles, had been blown down like so many matchsticks. We could only speculate that the tornado lifted a little before it hit us, or that in approaching our small island it had picked up enough water to reduce the velocity of the wind.

We continue to say our thanks.

GRIZZLY ENCOUNTERS ON THE CLARKE AND THELON RIVERS

Mel Baughman

TANDING HIGH ABOVE THE CLARKE RIVER, a tributary to the Thelon in Nunavut, we gazed across the valley at the crystal-clear, braided river clogged by packed snow. Grayling dimpled the surface of a backwater pond. Tundra rolled to the distant horizon. Small groves of black spruce huddled along the river. But what were those diggings in the hillside some two miles away? Curious and with time to explore, we paddled across the river and hiked up the side canyon. A half-dozen grizzly dens of various ages pocked the hillside. The most intact was egg-shaped, about six feet deep and three feet high and wide. Surely those were claw marks on the ceiling! Knowing that grizzlies don't oc-cupy their dens in midsummer, we felt perfectly safe but were mindful of their presence.

A few days later three of us hiked along an esker near camp while our fourth crew member, Paul, walked a half mile to a tun-dra pond to look for waterfowl. From our distant vantage point we spotted a grizzly feeding on vegetation in a patch of wet tun-dra across the pond from Paul. As it grazed through willows at the end of the pond less than two hundred yards away, Paul made a hasty retreat toward camp to avoid a close encounter. The next morning we returned to the willow patch to photograph the fresh grizzly tracks. Thereafter tracks appeared on nearly every sandbar along the river—and such bars were common on the Clarke and Thelon rivers.

We had a twelve-gauge shotgun with us but routinely left it in the canoe or at the campsite when we took hikes. Its purpose was to protect our food supply on this twenty-four-day trip. We didn't anticipate using it for personal protection.

The Ursus Islands on the Thelon were named for the grizzly (*Ursus horribilis*) that roam the islands' willow thickets and ponds. The river corridor we had traveled for nearly three weeks was prime grizzly habitat, so we didn't mind camping one evening on the tip of an island in this cluster. The hundred-yard-wide sandbar would give any grizzly ample opportunity to spot and avoid our campsite near the water's edge.

From this campsite we noted a high hill across the river and decided to hike to the top the next morning if the weather was reasonable. Fortunately, the rain that had fallen for the last week had stopped by morning, so we trekked about two miles up to the highest point. We could see for miles in every direction over the Thelon valley, as well as up the Tammarvi River. Once again caribou eluded our sight, but we spotted a moose about two miles away near some willows. Below us an animal swam across a tundra pond, probably a beaver or moose, we thought. From that distance, all we could detect was a dark-colored creature creating a wake.

On the hike downhill to our canoes, I drifted apart from the others to look for peregrine falcons around a cliff face. Sure enough, I spooked a falcon, which soared above the rocks. Turning away from the cliff, I caught motion out of the corner of my eye. Casually turning my head, I saw a grizzly fifty yards away walking near the rock pile. It hadn't spotted me yet. It occurred to me that this must be the animal we had seen a half hour earlier swimming across the pond far below. Should I lie down and hide or keep walking to put more distance between me and the beast before it saw me? On the pathway it was following, the grizzly would cross my scent line soon and know I was nearby. Keep walking! I reached for the telephoto lens dangling in a case from my belt and began to change lenses as I moved away. But I had taken just a few steps before the grizzly turned its head in my direction and stopped. Then it charged.

The grizzly covered ten yards in a few loping bounds, but stopped at a distance of forty yards. We stared at each other for several seconds, but I didn't move a muscle. This wasn't a conscious decision; I was just petrified with fear. Later I read that a lone male grizzly on the open tundra feels threatened at a threshold distance of fifty yards. This encounter could have gone either way. My immediate thought was, "Isn't it interesting how quickly a person's life can change? I could be badly mauled or killed in the next minute." But the barren-ground grizzly turned and ran up and over the rocky hill.

My heart started beating again, and I noticed that I hadn't changed lenses yet on my camera. Just then, Paul ran over to me. He'd been standing a hundred yards away and had seen the grizzly striding uphill. He had shouted to warn me, but the strong wind drowned out his voice. Feeling bolstered by Paul's presence and the fact that the grizzly had run off, we walked slowly toward a cleft in the hill where the grizzly had disappeared. Reaching a good vantage point, we saw the grizzly a quarter mile away, running hard across the tundra. We watched it until it was at least a mile away, still on the run.

Our last campsite of the trip was on a sandy bank among willows where the Thelon enters Beverly Lake. I counted thirteen piles of bear scat within a hundred yards of our tents, but this was where we were to meet our pilot for the flight out, because the deep water and sand beach would accommodate a floatplane. I didn't sleep well that night.

As the single-engine Otter rose into the sky the next day, I glimpsed a large, brown mammal in the willows near camp. Was it a grizzly or a musk ox? I'll never know.

EDITOR: *Luckily, this is the way most bear encounters end; however, if you are traveling in bear country you must be prepared to actually encounter bears. Personal protection (such as pepper spray), traveling in large groups, and understanding the signs of bear activity are all things you can plan for while organizing a trip. But it still takes considerable effort not to become complacent when paddling in areas where bears are active. This is always risky because bears—especially grizzlies—are simply too unpredictable. As the outfitter said when selling pepper spray to a paddler headed to bear country, "If this don't work, you just bring it on back, you hear?"*

UP THE CREEK WITHOUT A CANOE
Jack Stefanyk

ADVENTURE, CHALLENGE, EXCITEMENT. These were some of the words used by the college- and career-aged group from one of the Saskatoon churches that had showed up to hire the guiding and outfitting services of our camp. There were three young men and four young women, all rookie paddlers excited to be in the wilds of northern Saskatchewan for a ten-day canoe trip. As we sat around the lodge on the first day, they sized up some of the maps we had on our wall. Having done all the trips within ready reach of the camp, I was anxious to explore new territory and steered the discussion toward some routes that hadn't been done before. They were an eager bunch and didn't really know what they were getting themselves into—nor did I, as it turned out.

Looking at the map, we thought there might be a route via some small lakes, and with considerable bushwhacking, from the Sandy River across to the Paull River (these rivers are just north of the Churchill River, near Black Bear Island Lake). I had been on the Paull before, a small, picturesque river that is usually accessed by plane. The thought of getting there by paddle rather than plane, and thus saving money while "going where no man has gone before," was all the challenge we needed.

Because the group was small, I chose to go alone as guide, cook, and travel agent. The trip from Nemeiben up to Black Bear Island Lake was a breeze. It was familiar territory, campsites were plentiful, and with good weather, everyone was having a great time. But as we left the familiar confines of the Churchill behind and entered the Sandy, things began to change.

The first part of the Sandy was fun—lots of wading and poling as we journeyed upstream. But as we progressed farther upriver, the fun faded. After a long afternoon of pulling and dragging our canoes, we were ready to stop for supper and an early rest. But the campsite we were looking for never appeared. The river had become a never-ending maze of moose pasture—reedy, mosquito-infested marshland. There wasn't even a place to stop to build a fire for our supper.

I tried to appease the group's mutinous spirits with granola bars and old canoeing stories, but they weren't buying it. I now knew what Moses felt like. By 10 p.m. we were entering the twilight zone and feeling desperate. No one was talking and the "are we almost there yet" jokes were long forgotten. We paddled on. Finally, we spotted a campsite on a little rocky island about a hundred feet long by twenty feet across, with enough shrubs at one end to give us a little bathroom privacy. While the rest of the crew pitched tents, I quickly cooked supper, thanking my lucky stars that this tiny island had appeared when it did.

This was in the days of the old A-frame tents that needed to be pegged down at the corners—an impossibility on our lump of rock. The three guys slept in one such tent and the four women in another. A married couple, Ron and Joy, had one of the new freestanding tents. While I was cooking I noticed some low, black clouds rolling in from the west. They looked like huge feathery pillows, hanging so low they almost touched the tops of the scrawny spruce that dotted the landscape. I had never seen such a formation of clouds before, and they did not bode well for us.

I knew something was on the way, so we hurried through our meal and escaped to the tents just as the first raindrops began to fall. Within minutes, hail, wind, and rain like I'd never seen before poured down on our little island. Because it had been a long, hard day with good weather, the group assembling the tents had skipped putting on the rainflies and anchoring the guide ropes with large rocks. We paid for that mistake dearly.

Within seconds the guys' tent, with us inside, was flattened. There was absolutely no place to go, no place to hide. As we sat hunched under our nylon shroud, I was thinking that this was one of the most bizarre situations I had ever been in. Then I heard the shrill yell of one of the women from the other tent; above the storm, I heard something about canoes in the water.

It was now totally dark except for flashes of lightning, which lit the sky all around us. I peeked out to see that two of our aluminum canoes had been blown onto the river from their perches atop the island. I could also see that the women's tent was in the same shape as ours, but they had had the sense to take shelter in the freestander with Ron and Joy.

Being the leader of a trip like this had its advantages: respect, admiration, young female clients who I was sure thought I was cool. But there were also drawbacks, and this was one of them. Here I was in my shorts, soaking wet, lightning flashing so close you could feel it, hail as big as marbles pelting down on us, and now the canoes were floating toward the rapids we had just finished lining up about two hundred feet downstream. Someone—presumably the leader—needed to rescue those canoes before they were lost for good. So, seminaked and yelling at Ron to join me, I jumped in one of the two remaining canoes and set off by the light of the storm. Praying that we wouldn't be lightning rods, Ron and I managed to secure the two strays and tow them safely back.

And then, amazingly, the storm ended as quickly as it had begun.

We erected our flattened tents and spread a rolled-up and still semidry sleeping bag over one of the sopping tent floors. That was our bed for the night. On any other night, that might not have been satisfactory, but being thankful just to be alive makes discomfort a little easier to swallow.

EDITOR: *Conducting a canoe trip while maintaining continuous safety awareness is difficult when the responsibility for the group rests solely with the guide.*

GAIL, LEE, AND BEAR MAKES THREE

Lee Pearson

FEW YEARS AGO, MY WIFE AND I began a trip on the Nahanni, in the Northwest Territories, a trip we had long anticipated. Gail had undergone a kidney transplant nine years before, and since then we had been making annual canoe trips as a substitute for travel to exotic lands, which could threaten her suppressed immune system. We usually traveled as a couple rather than in a group, and only after I researched each trip carefully to avoid potentially dangerous situations. With this in mind, we started our Nahanni trip just north of Island Lake rather than attempt the rapids from Moose Pond.

The charter pilot we hired said he could land on a small lake to save us the long portage from Island Lake to the river. Prior to takeoff, he gathered some gravel and stones in a small box. Unusual behavior, but he was an experienced pilot, so I thought no more of it. The pilot flew his twin-engine Otter at high altitude to avoid the thick smoke blowing in from forest fires in Saskatchewan. As it turned out, ours was the only party able to fly in for several days due to the smoke cover. Our pilot cruised low over the tiny lake where we were to land and dropped the rocks from the window. What is this, I thought, some bizarre ritual to appease the water gods? In fact, as he later explained, it was to help him distinguish the water surface from the air above.

We landed successfully, noticing on touchdown a huge black bear at the other end of the lake. We're always delighted to spot wildlife but were surprised that it didn't run away at the sound of the engines: in our experience, bears are afraid of humans. I soon forgot about this sighting in the excitement of being in Nahanni country after the long planning and anticipation.

Our pilot left and we set up camp. With twenty-four hours of summer daylight, we didn't retire until nearly three in the morning. We simply covered our gear with a tarp, as we were only going to be there a few hours. Exhausted, we quickly fell asleep.

At 8:30 a.m. I awoke to find myself in a sitting position, as the window end of our small tent was being pushed in by something. When I instinctively elbowed whatever it was, it felt as if I had jammed my arm into a large rock. Instantly wide awake, I unzipped the tiny triangular window and looked out into the face of a black bear—just six inches from my own. Its bad breath and my own fear made me recoil.

Gail and I scrambled out of the tent, yelling and making ourselves as tall as possible. Thankfully, the animal left, although reluctantly. As we watched the bear retreat slowly into the bush, I told Gail that the bear was probably just curious.

We began to break camp, and I noticed dripping bear spittle all over the end of our tent. I was wondering aloud whether a small tear was the result of a tooth or a claw when Gail impatiently urged me to stop musing and get packing. What a great way to start a trip, I thought.

Our calm vanished as the bear reappeared, growling as it charged toward us. Both Gail and I instinctively picked up baseball-sized rocks and began throwing them in its direction. It kept coming despite several of these missiles bouncing off its head. We were retreating closer to the lake and considering a swim in the forty-degree water when the bear stopped fifteen feet from us and abruptly turned back into the woods.

"It was only trying to scare us," I told Gail matter-of-factly.

"Well it worked," she answered.

She also admitted later that running through her mind was

the disquieting idea that there were still eighteen days left in the trip.

We quickly loaded our canoe, to the sound of the bear thrashing around in the woods. Once we were a hundred feet from shore, Gail remarked that she was sure she would never walk again as her legs seemed to have turned to jelly.

I learned three valuable things from this experience:

- always sleep where baseball-sized rocks are available
- always have a two-door tent (for quick exits)
- don't test your bear spray until completely out of the tent

As word of our experience spread along the river, we became known as the Bear People, a tribute we could have done without. We encountered no more bears the rest of the trip, and Gail and I still go canoeing—although she sleeps very lightly. We now always keep bear spray and bear bangers on hand, and we sing and whistle our way through the woods to announce our presence.

EDITOR: *Bears are unpredictable. Planning for travel in bear country should include training in whatever personal protection you feel comfortable with, whether bangers, bear spray, or guns. It should also include contingency plans for as many different bear encounters as you can imagine. Throughout your trip do your best to be vigilant, and stay tuned to the signs of bear activity around you.*

MEETING THE BIG WHEEL AT THE WHEELER
Laurel Archer

N THIRTEEN YEARS OF CANOE tripping together, Brad and I had dealt with only one bear in camp. But when we did, it was a big one, and it didn't go away—we did.

Paddling the Geikie River in northern Saskatchewan one fine June day, we decided to check out the grayling fishing on the Wheeler River, which flows into the Geikie about thirty kilometers from Wollaston Lake. We dropped off our gear at a great campsite below the last rapid on the Wheeler and headed off to fish.

After a couple hours catching pretty little gray fish, we stopped at a lake that looked like it might harbor a few trout. Sure enough, we were successful trolling for a dinner-sized trout. It was getting late, so we started back to camp, looking forward to a good meal and a good night's rest.

But when we got back we discovered that someone had been using our camp to prepare lunch. The cooks had dumped fish guts and carcasses over the edge of the sand embankment in front of the campsite. While checking for any offal on land, we came across fresh bear sign.

We weighed our options. Maybe this *wasn't* such a good place to spend the night. On the other hand, it was getting dark and the mere prospect of honey mustard–baked trout made our stomachs rumble. We decided to stay. We built a fire, made supper, and erected the tent. Finally, we laid down our slightly sunburned limbs, taking a moment to admire the view down the channel. Marvelous. We quickly fell asleep.

Early the next morning, great splashing sounds below the sand bank awakened me. Then a twig snapped, and another. Looking out of the "viewfinder" presented by the tent vestibule, I expected a pleasant view of the mist hanging over the silvery waters of the Wheeler. Instead, my eyes focused on two ears atop the head of a big black bear. With a fish carcass clamped in its jaws, the head rose up over the bank, followed immediately by a gigantic body. Then the eyes came level with mine, framed by the tiny tunnel of blue and yellow nylon. The tent vestibule didn't allow me to judge the bear's size accurately, but I was convinced of its size when I shook Brad and exclaimed, "There's a *very large bear* looking at me!"

But the bear had already walked out of my limited view. Brad, not at all appreciating the shaking I was giving him, pulled the top of the sleeping bag off his head and groggily peered around.

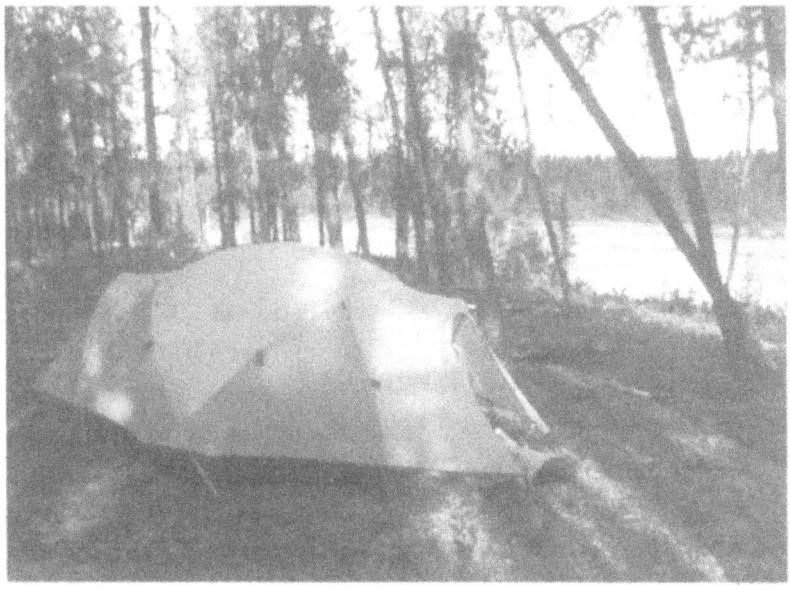

Campsite on the jack pine bench.

Clang! Clang! Our visitor was thoroughly investigating our metal environmental stove.

"I believe the *very large bear* that stuck its head in the tent door is now more interested in the kitchen than the bedroom," I said.

Brad mumbled something about unwanted houseguests as he wrestled on his red long underwear and crawled out to shoo the home wrecker on his way. Still rummaging for clothes, I could hear what sounded like the bruin using the stove grate for a toothpick. "Better that than chewing our plastic food barrels to bits," I thought.

As I was about to unzip the mosquito netting to step out, the infernal banging stopped. "Ah," I thought, reassured. "Brad's presence scared off the bear." Just then, I heard several thumps. Halfway out the tent door, I heard footsteps coming my way— fast. Zipping past the vestibule was a red blur: Brad hoofing it at high speed.

"What's happening?" I shouted as I jumped out. Looking left, I saw Brad standing with a log in one hand. Looking right, I saw the bear nonchalantly looking at Brad. Then the beast lay down, apparently bored.

Brad brandished his piece of jack pine, wild-eyed: "I was throwing pieces of firewood at it, and I accidentally hit it. It turned on me!" he explained. "Really!" he added.

"Oh," I said doubtfully, looking at our lounging guest, who was now picking nits off its fur.

"It turned on me, and—and then it lay down!" Brad continued.

The situation was unnerving. The bear—clearly the local Big Wheel—was completely at home right here at our campsite, where it had come for a nice lunch the day before. I didn't want to think about its *next* meal.

It was only five in the morning, but we decided it was way past our checkout time. We shoved the tent in the canoe, poles still in the sleeves, and threw our gear in on top. Ursus Major watched our preparations with a yawn. We still had to get it at least slightly away from our barrels, stove, and booties. The booties wouldn't have been much of a loss, but we couldn't leave without the food in those barrels.

We yelled, jumped around, and threw rocks. Finally, the bear deigned to move from the kitchen to the back patio. Then it scratched an ear, yawned, and lay down again in a spot of sunshine. We scurried around, one eye on the bear at all times, picking up the rest of our stuff.

Ready to go at last, we looked back one more time. The bear was chewing on the piece of firewood Brad had hit it with. We paddled on to Wollaston Lake, determined to avoid denning up at popular fishing spots forevermore.

EDITOR: *This bear story could just as easily have had a tragic rather than an unsettling end. By choosing to stay at the campsite after realizing it had been visited by a bear, Laurel and Brad were probably too complacent and not proactive in assuring their safety. You simply have to plan as best you can, make sure you have the equipment you need, know how to use it, and site your camp well with respect to your canoes so you can deal with new circumstances with the greatest number of options.*

THE WILD NAHANNI

Pam Little

M Y FRIEND SHIRLEY HAD BEEN a guide on the South Nahanni for many years, and after seeing her photos of that
beautiful, clear water I was determined to go there one day.
Shirley had described the rapids from Moose Ponds as some of
the most enjoyable she'd ever paddled.

My chance finally came, though: I would accompany a Parks
Canada expedition, which included the chief park warden and
three other wardens from Nahanni National Park Reserve. One
of these men was the first native person from Nahanni Butte to
paddle the Nahanni from the headwaters. My partner was Don,
a warden from Banff National Park. Ken and Rob were in the
second canoe, and Carl and Fred in the third.

There was still a lot of snow around in July when we flew into
Moose Ponds, even though the weather had been mild, even hot,
the week before our trip. We paddled out and camped on a beautiful gravel bar. That night it began to pour. In the early hours of
the morning I thought I could hear water and got up to have a
look. The rain, along with melt from the recent hot weather, had
made the river rise dramatically, and water was already lapping
into our kitchen.

The rain continued, and as we proceeded downriver that day
we realized that the big rapids we were paddling were normally
just small ripples, not even marked on the map. We all began to
worry just a little. The first marked rapid we came to was Initia-

tion Rapids, and we soon found ourselves paddling class 3 rapids through the trees along the side of the river. The main river channel looked horrendous.

Because many rapids were simply too big and too powerful to run, for the first couple of days we tried to line as many rapids as we could. Lining often involved wading with the canoe in waist-deep, moving water through thick willows far from shore. We were forced to approach Hollywood Rapids at the outside bend of the river. The place to portage would have been the lower side of the river on the inside of the curve. However, the river was so big and powerful at this point that we couldn't even go across. Thus began a four-hour portage that involved hauling all the canoes and equipment up the steep bank, walking around the rapid, and belaying people, canoes, and gear back down the bank to the river.

We still had to get across the river, and by now we were all a little freaked out. It was one of those places where you look at your partner and then at the raging river, knowing that you have no choice except to make this ferry. How could this have happened? Here I was, sitting at the edge of a wild river I had long wanted to paddle, facing a life-and-death situation none of us had expected.

Don and I made the ferry, as did Ken and Rob. But there was little time to enjoy our accomplishment. In the third canoe, Carl and Fred were probably too inexperienced for these conditions, and perhaps they even thought we were overly conservative by lining and sneaking down the edge of the river. I don't think they understood how big the rapids were and how powerful the current was. They capsized. The rest of us leaped into action and had a dicey time getting them to shore. After that swim, however, we *all* realized the gravity of our situation.

We continued downriver, finally arriving at Virginia Falls, where we met a party from a Nahanni River guide company. They had been waiting there for five days for the water level to drop. I think they were pretty frightened by what they saw when they first flew in and, exercising good judgment, they decided to wait for conditions to improve.

A boardwalk along the river here was built to serve the tourists who come in by floatplane to view the falls. When we arrived, the boardwalk was completely underwater. I couldn't even imagine how high the water must have been a few days earlier.

After the portage around Virginia Falls, we prepared to continue our trip. The guided group was happy to have another party with them for support. We all set off on a big ferry across the first canyon. The river was huge, with enormous waves. Partway across, one of the guides and a client capsized. Don and I were able to pull the paddlers to shore, but the canoe got away.

Ken and Rob pursued the canoe and managed to secure it. They clipped a throw bag to the capsized canoe, hoping to tow it to shore. There was enough rope in the throw bag for Ken and Rob to get to a small eddy at the edge of the river before the swamped canoe pulled the rope taut. Rob reached for a small tree in the eddy, and Ken jumped out, just as the throw-bag rope took up the full load of the swamped canoe in the powerful current. Instantly, Rob, the canoe, and the tree were torn from the eddy and went careening downriver.

In retrospect, I can say that this was one of the funniest things I've ever seen, but at the time it wasn't at all amusing. Rob was alone in the bow, being pulled rapidly downstream as Ken watched helplessly from shore. We shouted encouragement as Ken ran along shore after Rob and the canoes. The situation was saved by two other canoes in an eddy farther downriver. They managed to get the swamped canoe to shore, rescue Rob, and reunite him with Ken, who took a lot of ribbing for that episode.

The river was much more sedate after that, and we finished the trip with no further mishaps. The water level made canoeing much more dangerous than we had anticipated. I still hope to return to the Nahanni one day to run the river as it should be—clear water, pleasant rapids, and relaxed paddling.

EDITOR: *Planning for changing river conditions can be a tricky proposition. It is sometimes impossible to determine what drastic changes in water level will do to conditions, or even to know what influence conditions upriver will have where you are. Plan the best you can, inquire about local conditions, and make risk assessments based on the available information, including the skill levels within your group. Then be vigilant and make new decisions along the way if conditions deteriorate.*

ADVENTURE IN THE NIGHT

Doug McKown

N A JULY AFTERNOON, I WAS LEADING a group of twenty-six army cadets and eight instructors on a canoe outing down the shore of Lake Minnewanka in Banff National Park in Alberta. It was a breezy day on the large mountain lake, and it took about an hour and a half of hard paddling to reach the remote lakeside campsite. We were the only group in the large wooded campsite that evening, but it still required considerable organization to get everyone settled in for the night. Finally, everyone was in their tents, and silence descended.

During the night, I was awakened by shouting outside my tent. Amid the commotion created by sleepy instructors and excited cadets, I finally determined that a black bear was wandering around somewhere in our campsite. The instructors managed to shepherd all the cadets down to the lakeshore without actually encountering the bear.

Leaving two instructors to guard the cadets, the rest of the instructors and I headed back to deal with the bear. We were not in a good position. I was belatedly realizing that we were in a remote campsite, with no bear deterrents on hand, no contingency plans, and the potential for serious injury. However, we armed ourselves with pots and pans and, feeling reasonably secure in our numerical superiority, we advanced into the darkness of the trees. We could hear the bear moving around, but few things are harder to see than a black bear at night in the woods.

When we finally located the bear, it was in no hurry to leave the area, which wasn't good news: if a bear is not easily frightened away, it can become dangerous. This bear seemed to have become habituated to campsites, probably because it found them to be productive foraging sites.

With lots of shouting and pot banging we were finally able to drive the bear away. We set up a watch for the rest of the night, but luckily the bear never returned. When we finished the trip, I reported the incident to the warden service. They told me that a little farther along the lake, the same bear had kept two campers hostage up a tree for six hours the day following our adventure.

EDITOR: *This was a bad situation all around. In this case, my pretrip planning failed to include contingency plans for dealing with a bear. I think that, subconsciously, I dismissed the possibility of a bear encounter because the group was so large and likely to be making enough noise to discourage bears from approaching. Never a good assumption.*

FOSTER RIVER BURNOUT

Doug McKown

T HE WEATHER HAD BEEN HOT AND DRY all season, but this wasn't much cause for concern since it was not uncommon to see as many as a hundred forest fires burning at any one time during a hot northern Saskatchewan summer. Five days into a trip on the Foster River, we camped on a beautiful rocky point in the narrows of the lake, when we had our first glimpse of an active fire. It appeared as a tall plume of smoke on the horizon, resembling the mushroom cloud of a distant nuclear explosion. The fire lay in our general direction of travel but was still relatively far away.

The next day was breezy, and the forest fire was definitely getting bigger and appeared to be creeping closer to our line of travel.

Approaching a large fire like this, all you can hope for is to wind up on the upwind side, preferably on a large lake. The end of our paddling day at least put us on a wide area of river, although we still faced four or five kilometers of river and several rapids before Eulas Lake, the last lake on the Foster River.

The fire was close now. A billowing mountain of smoke blew toward us, heavy with black smoke rolling downwind over our heads. The fire was now directly in our path. We camped with some trepidation on a rocky point, just upstream of the next rapid. We knew this narrow piece of river would not be a good place to be trapped if the fire closed in. The smoke made the day as dark as a moonless night, with only a small strip of blue

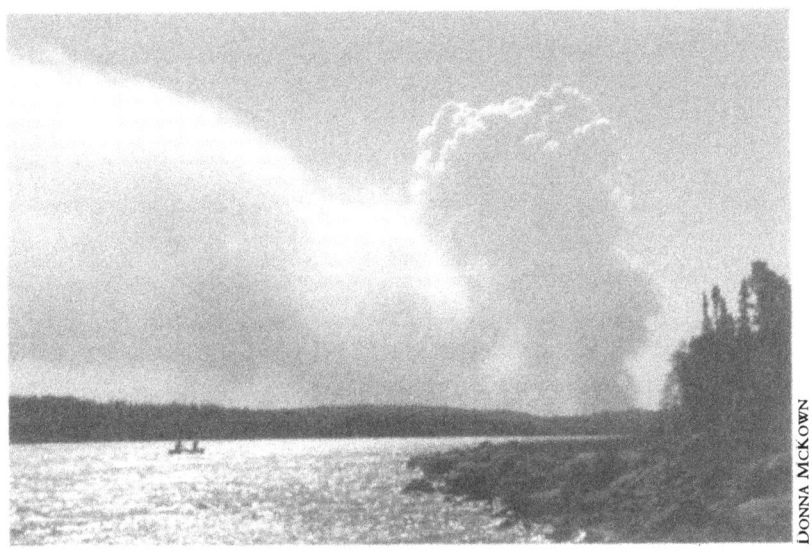

We were definitely getting closer to the fire.

sky along the horizon hinting at the sunshine above.

As we cooked our evening meal, we could sense the wind veering more directly toward us. Ash and burned spruce needles began to fall, settling on us like a blanket of black snow. If the fire kept moving forward, it would take only a spark or two to ignite our tents. As dusk fell, we heard wolves howling in the distance. Eventually, the wind died for the evening. Forest fires also tend to settle down at night, and we went to sleep hoping conditions would improve by morning.

We awoke to find less wind but more smoke. We decided to head downriver, running the rapids, in the hope we would be able to see the actual extent of the fire when we got to Eulas Lake. As we approached the lake, both banks were on fire. A brisk wind was blowing, and hot spots were bursting into flame as we paddled by. The entire east side of the lake as far as we could see was rumbling and seething with smoke so thick that general visibility was severely limited. We headed down the west side of the lake, hoping to skirt the edge of the flames.

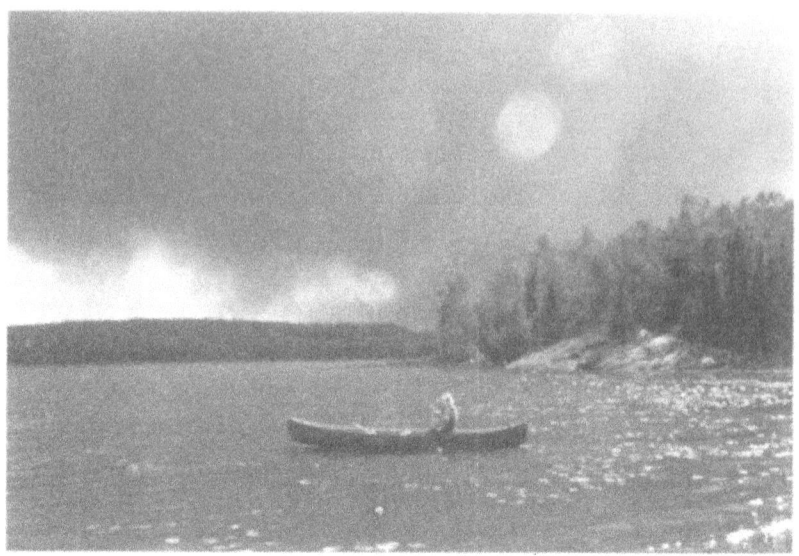

Our last campsite, very close to the fire.

We soon came to a narrows where an island sat only a couple hundred meters from the east shore. There was an out-camp fishing lodge on the island, and as we were passing by, a helicopter flew low overhead on its approach to the lodge. Spotting our canoes, the pilot waved us to shore and then landed on the island. We paddled to the dock at the lodge, relieved to encounter someone who was in a good position to tell us the extent of the fire.

The fire management officer in the helicopter indeed had the goods: we had paddled right into the middle of the biggest of the 285 forest fires in the region. Apparently, the entire forest surrounding the lake was in flames, cutting off the route we were taking. While the workers set up sprinklers and pumps to try to save the lodge, the officer agreed to radio an aircraft charter company to pick us up. The charter company had evacuated the residents of the lodge the day before we arrived, but we held out the hope that we could be shuttled downstream to the Churchill River so we could continue our trip from there.

The helicopter took off, leaving us on the island to wait for the plane, which would have to land on water mostly obscured by thick, dark smoke. We watched as the fire roared up the ridges just across the lake from us, the blaze crowning in enormous walls of fire along the heavily treed ridges. As the wind pulled this way and that in response to the fire, the lake basin would periodically fill completely with thick smoke before a breeze would whip through, clearing the smoke and raising our hopes that a plane would actually be able to land.

After three hours of anxious waiting, a twin Otter finally roared over the island. We quickly loaded our gear into the plane and took off into the smoky sky, flying along the upwind side of the fire, which was even more impressive from the air. The wind had originally blown the fire into a long, thin line, but a shift brought the flames toward Eulas Lake in a wall that stretched sixteen kilometers.

As our altitude revealed the enormity of the blaze all around us, we knew our canoe trip was done for. The pilot told us that the fire management center had ordered him to evacuate us to La Ronge. In the next few days the fire crossed Eulas Lake and began a march toward the Churchill River.

EDITOR: *Forest fires are a natural, regular occurrence. They can grow rapidly, travel incredibly fast, and change direction capriciously: never underestimate the danger of forest fires. If you encounter a forest fire, know what your options are and be prepared to move quickly. The problem, of course, is where to go. In many cases, all you can do is head toward the biggest, closest body of water and hope for the best.*

THE CAT AND THE RAPIDS

Jim Buckingham

DON'T KNOW EXACTLY how my friends decided that although it would be unwise for them to attempt to run a rapid with a large golden retriever in the canoe, it would be perfectly OK to run it with a cat in the boat. Bob and Bonnie regularly made weekend canoe trips on lakes with one or two golden retrievers, as well as one or two cats, in their canoe, but this trip on the Manigotogen River in Manitoba was different. It was a river trip with some really fun rapids, instead of the flatwater they were used to.

The plan was for Bonnie to walk the portage with the dog, while Terry, another paddler in the group, jumped into the bow seat to run the rapid with Bob. The cat was tied to the bow canoe seat with a leash so she couldn't get away. But it turned out that this cat, while calm during lake trips, became freaked out by the bouncing and splashing involved in running rapids. She was perched on the bow deck as the guys started into the rapid.

The best route lay close to shore, where a long, overhanging branch came within about ten feet of the canoe right at the top of the rapid. The cat evidently saw this branch as her last chance for freedom and made a frantic leap. Unfortunately, her leash was only about six feet long. She hit the end of the leash about four feet short of the branch and as she plummeted into the water gave a shrill death scream, which unnerved Terry not a bit. As the canoe went through the first few yards of the rapid he calmly put down his paddle, grabbed the leash, and coiled it like a deckhand on a ferry. The cat was dragged backward through the rapid, screaming like a banshee the whole way. Finally, the bedraggled, half-drowned cat was deposited in the bottom of the canoe.

After this minor interruption, the guys completed the rapid with style and grace—and right on line. The cat survived, but obviously with a renewed hatred of rapids.

EDITOR: *An amusing story, and fortunately one with a happy outcome, but taking animals along on a canoe trip requires careful organization to make sure that you are ready for any situation you and your pet may encounter. Animals can react to new situations in wildly unpredictable ways. They can capsize canoes, get lost, attract bears, create unnecessary distractions, play with porcupines, and bravely defend against skunks. Although they are thinking, active beings, animals have no "safety awareness." You must be very careful in predicting their reactions.*

CHAPTER FOUR

INJURY AND ILLNESS

ANY PEOPLE ASSUME that traumatic injuries are the most common dangers faced by canoeists, but physical injury is actually amazingly rare on canoe trips. Although most injuries are minor, blisters, scrapes, lacerations, sprains, and strains can still be troublesome. Trying to paddle all day after slicing your palm while cutting up vegetables can ruin your canoe trip and aggravate the injury.

Most traumatic injuries result from a decreased safety awareness resulting from laziness, complacency, inattention, fatigue, impatience, or carelessness. Maybe you tripped over a root and sprained an ankle during a portage, or drove an ax into your foot while cutting wood, or slipped while walking across a steep rock and broke your leg—the possibilities are endless.

Serious medical problems can occur with little or no warning. Difficult to deal with even under optimum conditions, such situations can be disastrous in the middle of a remote canoe trip.

During your pretrip planning, minimize the chances of illnesses developing by carefully inventorying preexisting health conditions and any medications each participant may be taking.

If an illness does occur, the impact can be reduced in two ways. The first is good preplanning. Having someone along on the trip who has advanced first-aid training is always a bonus. Before the trip, have an experienced physician or nurse help you assemble a comprehensive first-aid kit with a wide variety of treatments according to the level of training of your participants. Resources and training, coupled with a reasonable plan for evacuation along any point in your route, will allow the most options when illness or injury strikes. The second key to minimizing serious problems is early recognition: the sooner your safety awareness zeroes in on a developing illness, the better the chances for successful treatment.

I have been a paramedic for twenty years and have dealt with every kind of medical situation, but the consequences of fire seem the most terrible. First, many people overlook the hazards of fire on a canoe trip. It can happen so suddenly—campstoves that blow up, sparks and embers from campfires igniting, candles or cooking in tents, accidents with scalding liquids. Fire is a rapid, incredibly destructive force.

The technical outdoor clothing we wear now doesn't help, either: modern synthetics are incredibly flammable and burn rapidly and continuously, melting through skin and tissue. If you have ever seen the results of a pile jacket or nylon pants that melted and welded into skin, you would seriously consider returning to wool and cotton. And unless you have had one yourself, it's difficult to comprehend how painful and debilitating even a moderate burn can be.

Beyond the personal injury suffered in the fire, survivors have to cope with the immediate problem created by any loss of the clothing or equipment.

But, as always, the best defense lies in prevention.

If an illness or a traumatic injury does occur, your pretrip preparedness—having the appropriate supplies, understanding the level of training in your group, and knowing how and where to get help when you need it—will directly affect the success of the outcome.

THE HEART OF THE MATTER

Tom Brown

F IVE FRIENDS AND I, all experienced canoe trippers, were doing our first trip of the season in the northern part of Algonquin Provincial Park in Ontario. Ice-out had occurred just a few days earlier. With good weather in the forecast, we decided to extend our weekend trip by leaving early Friday morning and returning Monday morning.

We were on our own once we left behind the fishermen on the first few lakes, since few people venture into the heart of the park this time of year. The trip had gone well, and we were to spend our last night on North Tea Lake before heading out the next morning.

We were making our way down the lake late in the day. Spotting someone waving frantically at us up ahead on a point, we went over to investigate. A fisherman had come in to fish with a friend for the weekend, and he thought his friend was having a heart attack.

As I scrambled out of my canoe and headed for the tent, I tried to conjure up all the first-aid and CPR information I knew, although CPR would be of little use out here. Talking with the victim, "Eric," made it clear he was having heart problems and he needed to be evacuated as soon as possible, though he was unable to paddle or portage.

It was around 6 p.m., so we had only about two hours of daylight left. Paddling back to the access point for help would take roughly three hours. My group decided to lighten the load in one of the canoes and send the two strongest paddlers in it back to arrange for a plane the next morning. They would be off the river and through the portages before the light failed completely, but they would have to paddle across the last lake in the dark. Lights at the access point would help guide them out.

I sent two others of our group around the lake in search of wardens who would have radios, with instructions to return before dark. The last person remained with me to set up camp and prepare dinner. I returned to Eric to help make him as comfortable as possible and to let him and his friend, "Manuel," know what we were doing. There was a marked improvement in Eric's color once he heard we had a rescue plan under way.

The search for wardens turned up nothing, and in talking with other fishermen camped nearby, we learned that wardens probably hadn't been around that weekend. Eric's only hope lay with the canoe sent out to the access point.

I spent the night near Eric to keep my eye on his condition. He was very uncomfortable, and every time he sighed or moved I would bolt up to make another quick assessment of his condition. Neither of us got much sleep.

The sky didn't look very promising the next morning, with a low cloud ceiling. Despite the limited visibility, we still held out hope that a plane could make it in. About three hours after sunrise we heard an approaching plane, which we hoped would be the rescue plane. With the clouds almost down at treetop level, we were all anxious about the pilot's ability to identify our location, let alone land. But the plane came in low over the lake and landed right in front of our campsite.

Eric became so excited when he heard the plane that I became concerned. He got out of the tent by himself, and we actually had to slow him down and talk him into letting us help him to the plane. Eric and Manuel loaded on the plane, we began to pack up and then headed for home.

I called Manuel to learn how things turned out: Eric had suffered a full cardiac arrest minutes after reaching the hospital. Luckily, the hospital staff resuscitated him, and he survived. A few weeks later, a case of whiskey arrived at my doorstep.

Eric's survival was likely a result of lucky timing (our arrival on the scene) and our familiarity with the area and the local resources, which allowed us to develop and implement a rescue plan without delay. You won't always have incidents occur in a place you know this well, but your pretrip planning might save someone's life.

WHERE THERE'S FIRE, THERE'S FIRE
Doug McKown

WAS LOOKING AT THE RIVER, thinking that it would be hard
to imagine better canoe-tripping country than the Canadian
Shield on the east side of Lake Winnipeg in Manitoba. Our group
of four were relaxing on a large, flat granite ledge above the Pigeon River after a beautiful day of paddling. I was boiling water
over a small fire while Donna, my wife, started to clear the supper
dishes. Mary was preparing to put another loaf of bannock, our
food for the next day, in the reflector oven. The river ran deep and
smooth along the edge of the ledge, not two meters from where I

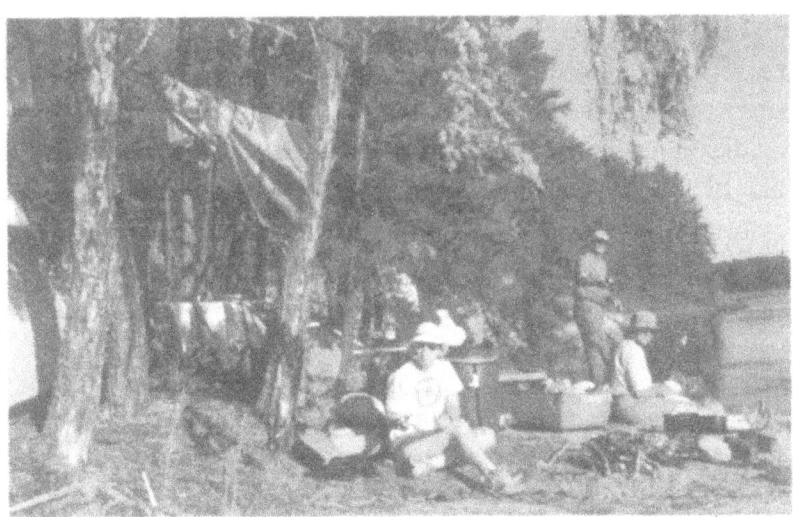

Our peaceful campsite minutes before the fire incident.

sat. I watched Jim at the other end of the rock, tending the reflector oven, as he baked the first loaf of bannock.

He had a large reflector rock set up, and a good little blaze was in progress. Reflector fires must be tended constantly to ensure that the oven is heated consistently, so Jim was standing in front of the fire, looking down and tapping logs into place now and then with his foot, as he always does.

I had just turned to talk to Donna when things began to happen very quickly. Out of the corner of my eye I saw Jim shuffling back from the fire, shaking his left leg. It took him another few seconds to realize what was happening.

"My pants are on fire!" he shouted, hopping frantically. The bottom of his left pant leg had ignited, and flames surrounded his ankle. Mary and Donna were frozen in horror, and Jim was still shaking his leg.

I shouted, "Hit the water!" As soon as the words were out of my mouth, Jim took two steps and dove straight into the river, the flames and smoke arcing as he went in.

In an instant the danger was over. Jim swam back to shore, climbed out, and we all gathered to assess the injury.

The lower twenty centimeters of his pant leg were gone, and there was a ten-centimeter burn on the outside of his leg, but that seemed to be the extent of the tissue damage. A little burn medication, some bandages to protect against infection, and regular dressing changes the rest of the trip, and Jim healed fine. Had he been just a few more meters from the water or had a few more seconds passed before he reacted, it could have been a debilitating injury.

EDITOR: *Accidents involving fire usually happen very quickly. Dealing with injuries must be part of your pretrip planning, but keep your safety awareness tuned in at all times to avoid potential injuries and, if they do happen, to contain the damage.*

THE LEMON THEORY WORKS

Tom Brown

E WERE ANTICIPATING A GREAT TRIP. We would be taking clients on a six-day canoe-tripping course in a beautiful, rugged, and remote area that none of us had traveled through before. In the previous week, the weather had changed from spring to summer, and hot, dry weather was forecast for the next few days.

We spent two days in base camp teaching canoeing and camping skills and trip preparation. All the usual trip planning activities went smoothly, but while reviewing medical forms, I discovered that one of the participants had recently been under a doctor's care for strep throat. Rob had also indicated that he was still taking antibiotics two weeks after the original diagnosis and treatment. He had forgotten to take some of his medication, so, instead of completing the course of antibiotics in the standard ten days, he would instead take seventeen days, finishing on the third day of the trip. He told me he felt fine and had been symptom free after the first day of medication. I mentioned this to the course director, but it didn't seem like something to worry about.

We split the group in two, with a party starting at each end of the route. We would meet in the middle and spend one night together before finishing. I was leading one group, and the course director took the other.

The first day went without a hitch. The weather was perfect— hot and sunny with almost no wind. The route was as rough as expected, though. The portages were overgrown and few had signs. On the second day we had a long portage to do, which would take much of the afternoon. Rob had unintentionally finished his prescription early by dropping the remainder of his medicine overboard while trying to take his noon dose.

It was hot, and the portage took a lot out of us. When I arrived at the end of the portage as the sweep person, two people were missing but accounted for: one of the student assistants had paddled with Rob out on the lake for a swim to cool off because Rob wasn't feeling well. We loaded up and went to meet them before setting off to find a campsite.

At camp, Rob went straight to bed, and it looked like his strep throat was back. The rest of us discussed the situation around the campfire that night. We knew we had to get Rob to a doctor. We decided to push on to meet the other group the next night. From that location we could paddle out to get help in about half a day. Rob was told of and agreed to the plan. With the group we also discussed how contagious strep throat is and reminded everyone not to share water bottles.

We awoke on the third morning to what would be the hottest day yet. We kept Rob's fever under control with over-the-counter painkillers from our first-aid kit and put him in a boat with one of the strongest paddlers. He had not eaten since lunch the day before and was now finding it hard to even drink water and juice. We knew we would have to pay close attention to prevent Rob from becoming dehydrated.

In the afternoon, the person paddling with Rob began to tire, so we switched boats. I jumped into Rob's boat, leaving all my gear in my own boat, including the maps. We had reviewed our progress at lunch and were doing well. Only a couple small lakes and short portages lay between us and the designated meeting point with the other group.

Rob was no longer able to paddle. He felt he could walk across the portages, but not much more. Toward the end of the afternoon we finally reached the next lake. It had taken us much longer than expected. I kept checking with the student leaders about our location, and they seemed confident that everything was OK.

But it just didn't look right. I finally retrieved my maps: all afternoon the students had been trying to make our location fit the map, a common problem when you are in the wrong place. Fortunately, I had brought topo maps, since we had been using the canoe route map for navigation, and was able to identify our current location. There were two creek and lake systems leaving the lake, and we took the wrong one. Preoccupied with Rob, and with my maps stashed in the other boat, I didn't notice the error.

The group was pretty discouraged because we all knew we would have to backtrack to get off this lake. We made camp for the night. The next morning it was clear that Rob was finished traveling. He needed to be evacuated.

We decided to wait for three hours, until 10 a.m., to see if we could attract the attention of the local air service. We never heard a thing, so two of the strongest paddlers set off to find the other group, alert them to the problem, and then continue on to get help. The rest of us waited all day with signal fires at the ready, but no planes came close.

Late in the afternoon I thought I heard a chopper, so I had the group light the signal fires. A few minutes later the provincial air ambulance appeared over the horizon. When it landed about a hundred meters from our campsite, we took Rob over. We passed all the paperwork to the paramedics, including our written history from the onset of the sickness. And then the chopper was off again.

The next morning we headed off to meet the other group. After an all-day paddle, we joined them at the campsite, two days late. That night another member of our group fell ill, and we realized he may have inadvertently used Rob's water bottle the first night Rob was sick. After breaking camp in the morning, the groups separated again, our group heading to the access point with the new victim, and the other group taking another route back.

We certainly had more than our share of lemons. Upon analysis, we found that many factors had contributed to this incident: hot weather, the unfamiliar area, the overgrown and unmarked portages, antibiotics not taken as prescribed, and people's sharing water bottles. And, of course, the navigational error that forced the emergency evacuation issue. If any one of these lemons hadn't been there, an air evacuation might have been avoided.

EDITOR: *When you are leading a group, all responsibilities fall on you. Do the best pretrip planning possible, and then be vigilant for the whole group for the duration of the trip. Don't underestimate the difficulty of keeping track of all the minor problems that develop on a trip, which may eventually develop into a larger problem. In a situation like this, good organization, proper planning, and ongoing evaluation of the situation allowed the trip leader to make the best of his opportunities.*

The problem of the students' trying to get the map to fit the terrain is sometimes called "bending the map," and unfortunately it afflicts experienced paddlers, as well.

BREAK A LEG

Doug McKown

T WAS THE ITCHING THAT WOKE ME UP; the new cast was
still wet. As I looked out the hospital window, I was surprised
to find that it was only early evening. The hospital was not where
I expected to end up when I left Banff early that morning.

I drove through the front ranges of Banff National Park in Alberta on the way to the Sheep River canyon, where a twisting,
rocky river flowed through rolling foothills. I was wondering
about the water level that our party of eight would find in the
river. Like most rivers in the foothills, the Sheep floods early, leaving little water for paddling by mid-July. However, it had rained
frequently over the past week. As I drove through the valleys
and hamlets, every stream was bursting its banks, flooding the
ditches and sloughs. Draining out of the mountains, this water
was all destined for the Sheep River canyon.

There was a great deal of activity as I pulled into the campsite
to join my friends. Tents were coming down and canoes were
being lashed to the tops of vehicles. In short order our little car-
avan was winding its way to the top of the canyon.

All worries about insufficient water were behind us—the report
from the ranger station confirmed that the river was indeed flowing high and fast from the recent rains. We normally paddle this
river at a flow of about 15 to 25 cubic meters per second. Today
the water was boiling along brown and turbulent at 77 cms.

I was paddling solo in my old red Tripper. Heather and Keith, and Bill and Lynn, were also in Trippers. The fourth boat was a Discovery 169 paddled by Bucky and his twelve-year-old daughter, Alison. Finally, there was Willie, paddling a short solo river canoe. All of us were experienced paddlers who, with the exception of Heather and Keith, had run the Sheep before. We were all looking forward to a day of exciting whitewater canoeing through a beautiful foothills canyon.

This section of the Sheep is winding and narrow, with boulders, ledges, steep canyon walls, impressive scenery, and nearly continuous rapids. The water roars through the canyon, creating chaotic waves that break and rise in an endless dance. At this water level the Sheep River is continuous class 3, with few breaks from the noisy rapids.

We pushed off into the swirling, rushing currents and spent the next two hours paddling, crashing through big waves, and catching fast eddies below steep chutes. Finally we stopped for lunch on a sunny ledge at the base of a tall cliff.

Everyone was having a great time, and we were soon on our way again. We changed leads, turned, and surfed, but always remained aware that we were responsible for one another's safety on such a hazardous river. We were well aware of the hazards. First, since all of us except Willie were paddling open canoes, swamping was a constant concern. Every wave and ledge splashed water into the canoes. The trick was to stop and empty the boats frequently enough to prevent swamping.

Another hazard was the unbroken run of rapids, coupled with steep canyon walls. This would have made it difficult to get out of the river or execute a successful rescue. Finally, since the foothills rivers begin high in the Rocky Mountains, the water usually remains dangerously cold year-round—an excellent incentive to stay upright.

When a day is going well, it is always a surprise when everything suddenly seems to go *wrong*. I had just come through a large set of standing waves. Using a little chute, I pulled into a small eddy on river left. Bucky was next, and he stopped on the other side of the river to empty his canoe. Heather and Keith followed, sitting very low due to water already in their canoe before they hit these last waves. They were in the center of the river, not able to maneuver quickly with the water's extra weight. They tried to turn toward shore, but the canoe capsized as their weight shifted, and they were plunged into the cold, swift water.

I shouted "Boat over!" to alert the rest of the group. Bucky dove for his throw bag while I looked upstream to check on the others. Bill and Lynn were also having problems with a boat full of water, but it looked as if they would be able to struggle to shore on their own. Willie was still far upstream, unaware of the current problem. I pulled out into the current, paddling fast to catch up to the capsized canoe. At this point, the river was straight for about a hundred meters before making a sharp turn and plunging over a two-meter ledge beside a small chute.

Bucky shouted "Rope!" as he tossed the throw bag to Heather and Keith. Both paddlers had managed to hold onto their canoe and paddles, but only Keith was in a position to grab the rope. Bucky held tight as Keith struggled to hold onto the rope and the canoe. As current pressure built up on the capsized canoe, Keith's cold fingers lost their grip on the canoe. As he swung into shore at the end of the rope, I chased Heather and the canoe downriver. I grasped the end loop of the overturned canoe and made sure that Heather was unhurt and still able to help in this rescue.

The ledge was coming up fast and we were quickly running out of time. There was no time to perform a boat-over-boat rescue or even get Heather into my canoe. She held onto the end of her canoe as I used mine to nudge her boat out of the current and into an eddy above the ledge. Paddling hard, I was able to turn her canoe just as we approached the top of the ledge. The canoe was completely upside down, and Heather was safe in the eddy, held between the smooth cliff wall and the overturned boat. She was able to hang onto the cliff firmly enough to stay in place, but I wasn't so lucky. My canoe was still in the current, sliding backward toward the ledge. I reached for the overturned canoe, but my hands slid uselessly along the smooth plastic surface.

I knew that I was going over the ledge, so I pivoted the canoe around to fall sideways over the rough surface. It wasn't a big drop, and I was able to land upright with a strong brace. I was balancing quite well when the canoe filled with water and sank beneath me. The water was just as cold as I thought it would be. As I floated free of the canoe, my hands were already going numb.

So there I was in the water with my canoe below a tricky drop, with continuous class 3 rapids stretching down the canyon as far as I could see. No one was in a position to help me. How could this have happened?

The worst part was that I knew it wasn't over yet. I was actually in an eddy along the edge of the waves at the bottom of the ledge, standing on relatively smooth rock in virtually still water about a meter and a half deep. I held the end loop of my canoe as I debated whether or not I could make it to shore—if that would even do me any good. Shore was a fifty-foot vertical cliff.

As I stood there pondering, the canoe was sucked underwater at the edge of the eddy and floated past me, back upstream. The current then swung it out into the river, carrying it downstream again, a meter underwater. I instinctively grabbed the gunwale as the canoe came past. What I couldn't see was the rest of the canoe underwater. The end of the canoe hit the side of my right shin, pinning the inside of my right foot against a small ridge of rock. There I was, stuck between a rock and a hard place.

My leg moved, and I felt the bones in my right ankle break as I was swept off my feet into the turbulent rapids. The situation had definitely deteriorated: now I was swimming down a wild river with my canoe and a badly broken ankle. I tried to keep the canoe parallel to the current as I went under and through the continuously breaking waves. About a hundred meters into this frothing, swirling swim, Willie finally caught up to me. By then I was ecstatic to see anyone; however, since he had only his little solo canoe, I knew he wouldn't be able to get both me and my canoe out of the river. I released the canoe to his care, and off he went downriver.

Without the canoe I was able to swim a little more efficiently toward shore. After another hundred meters or so, I spotted a couple large boulders just offshore that didn't have too much water flowing over them. With careful aim, I was able to push myself onto the rocks, at last coming to a welcome stop. I still had my paddle, of course, and by using it for support I was able to clamber down to a little eddy below the boulders. I stood there, wet, cold, and wondering about my poor canoe. There was still no one in sight upstream. In a short while—it seemed like a long while to me—Bucky appeared, paddling solo. As he pulled into the eddy I jumped in and we charged off downriver in search of Willie and my canoe. While we paddled, he filled me in on what was happening upstream. Bucky had gotten Heather and Keith back together, put Alison in with them, and then headed down to find me. Bill and Lynn and Heather and Keith were paddling together, moving slowly and carefully.

Since Bucky and I were alone, we had to be particularly careful. Down the canyon we went, stopping once to flip the canoe over and empty it. We were beginning to wonder where Willie could be. The flooding river had filled the bottom of the canyon, leaving little but steep walls and swirling eddies. Finally, we came around a corner and spotted him sitting beside his canoe on the only exposed gravel bar we had seen all afternoon.

Beside him, looking somewhat worse for wear, was my poor canoe. Missing its deck plate, it had deep creases, a broken thwart, and two twisted gunwales, but the damage was mostly superficial. When the rest of the group caught up, I was able to paddle it to the take-out without further incident.

Now, lying in my hospital bed following the operation that

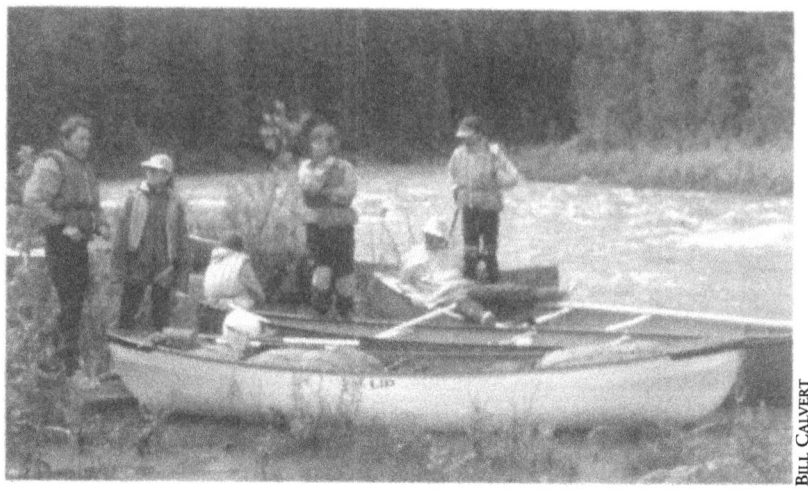

In my canoe, on the gravel bar where we finally caught up to the lost canoe.

left two steel pins in my ankle, I look forward to getting back into my canoe. What I remember most about this accident is the utter facility with which my bones were broken. The power of the current against the canoe was so strong that my leg might as well have been made of tissue paper.

Should this simple capsize have developed into such a serious accident? Probably not. It is always easy to make judgments after the event. I have fully repaired my canoe, and it has taken me on many enjoyable adventures since this accident occurred. All we can hope to do is survive and learn something in the process.

EDITOR: *Dangerous situations can develop quickly, even with solid planning. I like to think I could have reacted better, but split-second decisions were necessary. Luck, and the fact that we were only on a day trip, prevented this from becoming an even more serious situation.*

A FEVERISH TRIP ON THE GULL RIVER

Mel Baughman

N MINNESOTA WE HAD HEARD that the Gull River in neighboring Ontario was challenging to run because of rough water and overgrown portage trails, but the scenery, fishing, and whitewater thrills on twenty-four rapids were reputed to be worth the weeklong trip. Located just a hundred miles north of Thunder Bay, with good road access at both ends, we wondered why it didn't receive more canoeing pressure. An experienced trip leader I know had taken a group of Scouts down the river without much difficulty, so it couldn't be too rough. And the six canoeists in our crew were seasoned wilderness travelers with plenty of whitewater experience. During our trip planning, we made meticulous lists of food and equipment, and based on our considerable collective experience we felt prepared for whatever challenges the river held. We planned to paddle a leisurely seven miles per day for seven days to complete the fifty-one-mile trip, leaving plenty of time for fishing.

The first rapid gave us an adrenaline kick, which helped us push through the following three-quarter-mile portage over and around blown-down timber. The center thwart on my canoe broke on this portage, but we were able to replace it with a thwart from an abandoned canoe we found. Running two more rapids revived us, but we covered only four miles that first day.

The second day we paddled and portaged through four more rapids, making just three miles. Unusually high water flooded into the shoreline shrubs and created chains of big, standing waves. Several long, unrunnable rapids had no portage trails at all. We clung to the gunwales of our canoes and waded thigh deep over slippery, submerged boulders for hundreds of yards along the shoreline. No problem, we thought. This is a leisurely trip; we can make up for lost time later in the week.

Sure enough, the third day we negotiated four more rapids and covered seven miles. Encouraged by our faster progress, we camped early to fish at the confluence of a major tributary. With two fourteen-inch walleyes already dangling on our stringer, my paddling partner and I drifted around in an eddy, casting for more fish. Suddenly the water erupted at my side. A nine-pound northern pike had engulfed one of the walleyes and was thrashing on the surface. I grabbed a net and scooped up the big northern. We snapped photos for evidence of our encounter, then released the northern.

Shortly after a delicious fish dinner I felt a slight twinge of pain when I urinated. By next morning the unmistakable signs indicated that I had a urinary tract infection. Midmorning of day four, as we drifted through a pool, I told the group about the infection and asked that we paddle hard to get off the river by the next day so I could get medical attention before the infection worsened.

Years earlier, I routinely carried the proper medicine for this problem, but it had been so long since I'd had a UTI that I stopped carrying it.

For the rest of the day the river challenged us with rapids with high water, rough walking in the river, and tough portages. Mosquitoes, no-see-ums, and deerflies pestered us interminably. Did I mention that it rained all day? At the end of that grueling fourth day we had negotiated ten rapids and covered over nineteen miles. Exhausted, I went to bed right after dinner. My head ached, my body hurt, and I felt miserable from the infection.

The next morning we continued downriver through six more

rapids, including a mile-and-a-half portage. We reached the take-out bridge in late afternoon of the fifth day after paddling eighteen miles. We flagged down a passing car and paid the driver twenty dollars to take one of us to the van parked a dozen miles away.

Finally reaching Thunder Bay in the van, we checked into a motel for the night. Rather than seek medical attention at the local hospital, I decided to tough it out until we returned to Minnesota the next day. I didn't sleep well that night, making numerous trips to the bathroom. When I finally saw a doctor about five o'clock the following afternoon in St. Paul, my temperature registered 104.5 degrees. Another half degree or so and I might have gone into convulsions. Fortunately, tests indicated that the infection hadn't spread to my bloodstream, so I took the prescribed doses of antibiotics and fever medication, then went home. Within twenty-four hours I felt fine.

My biggest mistake was not getting medical attention at the first opportunity in Thunder Bay. I could have solved my problem faster and avoided a dangerous, potentially deadly, situation. I'm grateful to my fellow canoeists for sacrificing their vacation time to get me off the river quickly.

EDITOR: *Medical emergencies cannot always be foreseen. However, as part of your pretrip planning, ask each member in the group about existing medical problems, including latent conditions such as allergies, and ensure that members bring an adequate supply of medications for their conditions. Establish what the closest exit points are along your route, how to contact rescue resources, and how quickly you can evacuate someone. In the midst of an emergency, you will need to evaluate the situation as it unfolds and make appropriate decisions, such as waiting for outside help to arrive or evacuating the injured or ill person yourselves.*

BURNED

Tom Brown

I T WAS MIDSUMMER, THE HEART OF canoe-tripping season,
in Algonquin Provincial Park in Ontario. The park was busy
close to the access points, but I had been out for a week with
some friends, deep in the interior and away from the crowds.
We had just one night left to spend in the bush, on McIntosh
Lake, before returning home. An easy four-hour paddle the next
day would get us back to Canoe Lake.

It was getting late in the day and we were cruising the shoreline, looking for an open campsite. Up ahead we could see a
group camped at the next site. There seemed to be a lot of activity, but that wasn't unusual. When we got closer, though, it became obvious that something was wrong. One of the leaders,
"Michel," came down to shore to ask if any of us knew first aid.
We were all trained first-aiders and offered to help.

About fifteen minutes earlier one of the campers in their group
had dropped a pot of noodles that was too hot to touch, and it
had landed on another boy. Michel wasn't sure how serious the
burn was. The victim, "Thomas," was lying on his stomach with
the other counselor watching over him.

I wasn't expecting what I saw. Thomas had second-degree
burns on a significant portion of his back and down most of one
leg, but the counselors didn't seem overly concerned. I guess they
just didn't know how serious the situation was. This burn covered
over ten percent of Thomas's body—probably closer to twenty

percent. There were a significant number of blisters, many already broken. The counselors had done the right thing by getting Thomas's clothes off right away. The burn was cooling in the air, and with so many open blisters, further cooling with water was out of the question. Thomas was very pale and complaining of nausea.

I glanced at my watch: 5:10. I went back to the boat and told my group what the problem was, quickly putting a plan together to get help. We all knew we had to get this kid out of there that night.

I was working in the park at the time and knew most of the staff. In particular, I knew all the pilots and had memorized the phone number for the air base residence. I was hoping we would be able to catch someone at the base if we could get a call through in time.

With only about four hours of light left, we knew time was tight. Two members of my group would dump their gear here and paddle and portage out as fast as possible. They would head to Arowhon Lodge, where we knew there was a phone, and which was an hour closer than the Canoe Lake access point. This would leave a little over an hour of daylight to get a plane into the lake and then out to Huntsville.

We would also send someone back to Timberwolf Lake, where we had met two wardens earlier that day. We weren't sure if they were still there or if they had gone on to another lake or returned to their vehicle, which was parked nearby. This second canoe would search for the wardens and then return to us before dark if they were unsuccessful. Both rescue teams took with them the phone numbers of the pilots' base and residence and the camp, and everyone knew it was critical to get help that night.

I returned to Thomas with the remaining member of our group. We knew we would have to start to treat the shock as best we could. We told Thomas, who was just twelve years old, that help was on the way and that we would stay with him until a plane came. He was a little nauseated from the shock, but we tried to get him to drink some fluids. He was getting cool to the touch and beginning to shiver, so we used some clean space blankets to warm him. We continued to reassure the victim and encourage him to drink as much as possible.

Around 8 p.m. we finally heard a plane approaching. My partner signaled to it using a strobe we carry with us. The pilot landed the Turbo Beaver and came into the camp, leaving his helper on the plane. We quickly but carefully loaded Thomas into the plane. He would have to lie on the floor, as sitting was out of the question. The plane took off for Huntsville, where an ambulance would be waiting along with staff from the camp. The plane would have just enough time to get in before dark.

That evening, once all the campers were in bed, the remaining members of my group talked with the two counselors about the incident. They had basic first-aid training but not enough to deal with injuries in a remote setting. They hadn't realized how serious the burn was or that Thomas could have died from shock, and they hadn't researched how to get help if they needed it.

If you plan to spend significant time traveling away from civilization, wilderness first-aid training can help you assess situations that need immediate medical attention, those that need medical aid but not immediately, and those you can treat in the bush. In this case, the knowledge we had gained from canoe-tripping certification and from wilderness first-aid courses likely saved a life.

We learned later that Thomas was immediately sent by air ambulance from Huntsville to the special burn unit in Toronto. All the effort paid off, though, as he survived with very little scarring.

EDITOR: *This camping group was in serious trouble. They lacked the necessary knowledge to deal with the severity of the injury, and they didn't have a plan for how or where to seek help. A lucky encounter with Tom's group saved the boy's life, but proper organization and pretrip planning are requirements for every backcountry trip.*

A TRIP CUT SHORT IN NOOTKA SOUND

Dean McLeod

ONCE ACCOMPANIED A GROUP of juvenile-delinquent teenage girls on an eighteen-day sea-canoeing trip in November around Nootka Island on the west coast of Vancouver Island, British Columbia. These young people had significant personal and social problems but were able to keep up their health and spirits during that wettest month of the year. They loved the irony of finding, upon returning to their van at the end of the trip, that the music playing on the radio was "How I Love a Rainy Night."

While planning for the trip, the leaders had decided to bring along a small Swede saw and a Hudson's Bay ax so that even in the worst of weather they could get a fire going. The group leaders and participants alike became progressively more adept at choosing the best woods and wielding the small Swede saw. The ax, however, was considered more dangerous, both to the user and to someone else if an altercation occurred, so the teenagers were not allowed to use it. The leaders who split up the sawn wood used the utmost care in the continuously wet, slippery conditions.

The teens, of course, really wanted to use the ax. Eventually, one of them sneaked the ax away to split an armload of kindling. She only misjudged her timing once, but it was enough to cut her left index finger down to the bone.

We quickly dealt with the initial trauma of the injury but were then faced with what to do next. This was a serious injury.

The leaders held discussions among themselves, with the injured girl, and then with the whole group. Even if we had been successful in our attempt at cleaning the deep, wide cut, and even if the bandage held, we still faced the challenge of keeping the wound clean over the remaining ten days. If it became infected, we knew we couldn't easily care for a septic invalid. Now two hours after the accident, we came to the conclusion that the wound would require proper disinfecting and stitches in a hospital, likely followed by a course of oral antibiotics to knock out any infection.

We were eight days into an eighteen-day remote trip in rainy early-winter weather, by canoe, on the salt water of the Pacific Ocean. For reasons of social dynamics and gear storage we had chosen to have two people per canoe. Reviewing the situation, we realized how little margin for safety we had planned into our trip and how little room for error our skills, equipment, and situation afforded. At first light the next day, we would head back toward the last point of civilization we had encountered.

In November, all the lodges were locked tight, and the only vessels in the area were the twice-weekly ocean tugs that were unlikely, for navigational reasons, to stop long enough for some crazy canoeists to paddle out to the middle of the three-kilometer-wide channel. So if we saw, and could hail, a boat we would, but we assumed that the quickest, most reliable rescue was going to happen under our own steam.

The strongest leader teamed up with the injured girl, and we began a twenty-hour paddle over two days, en route to the Tahsis Hospital. Partway there, we approached the hamlet of Esperanza, noting on the dated map we had that it was, or had been, a hospital. It was not. But the group now in charge of the place was supportive: they ran the injured girl to the hospital in their own motorboat and put the rest of the wet, tired group up for the night.

It is always surprising how a relatively small injury can cut short a trip and also create logistical and organizational chaos in an instant.

EDITOR: *Everything changes once one of your party becomes ill or injured. This is when pretrip planning bears fruit. Try to plan for every possible situation, and have the resources available to treat and transport the victim.*

CHAPTER FIVE
THE CHOICES PEOPLE MAKE

ANOEING IS ALL ABOUT CHOICES: where to go, what to take, when to stop. In theory, more experienced paddlers make better choices; however, some paddlers still rely on the old adage, "It won't happen to me." But a simple misjudgment can lead to big trouble, so in that sense people can actually be the biggest hazard of all on canoe trips, particularly if you're traveling with a group. The fewer people in the group, the fewer people around to make mistakes, but this also leaves you with fewer resources and fewer options.

A variety of circumstances and conditions influence how a bad decision is made, which makes it difficult to generalize about how things may go wrong. Pretrip planning and organization should give you sufficient resources to deal with whatever situation arises. The best approach when you are actually in the field is to maintain a constant, focused level of safety awareness. Before acting on decisions, take the time to think through the likely consequences.

LEAP FOR LIFE

Doug McKown

HE KEEPER IS A SMALL RIVER that runs through the beautiful Canadian Shield country along the border of Ontario and Manitoba. My partner Jim and I were having a wonderful time paddling down a small lake toward the river's outlet. Our friends Donna and John were a few hundred meters behind us. I knew there was a short rapid at the end of the lake, but I was confident we could handle it easily. That should have been a clue that I was about to have a "stupid" day.

The river exited the lake through a rock garden and disappeared around a bend. We stopped at the top of the rapid, and I climbed out onto a rock to get a better view of the route. Since I couldn't see around the bend, I scampered down the shoreline to better see what was involved. The rock garden ended in a steep ledge, with a drop of about a meter. While not particularly dangerous, running the ledge with our loaded canoe might lead to a swamping, followed by an unpleasant swim down the rest of the rapid.

There was a large, flat rock just above the ledge where the current didn't look too fast, and I thought we could pull into the eddy just upstream. We could then line or lift the canoe over the ledge and be on our way. This seemed like a reasonable plan, so we waved to Donna and John and headed down the rapid. We maneuvered quickly through the rock garden, and I saw the flat rock approaching. But it seemed that the ledge was approaching even faster, and the eddy was looking smaller and smaller. Already committed, I angled the canoe toward the gap. When the moment arrived, I shouted, "Draw!" Jim dug in with his paddle, and I reached out to help bring the stern around. That was when we slammed into the rock. Not the big, flat rock, but the rock in the entrance to the eddy, hidden just under the surface. The rock I would have seen when I scouted the route if I had been paying better attention.

Although we instantly came to an abrupt halt, the canoe kept rotating as the current pushed us around. Then the canoe banged against the big, flat rock and slid backward toward the ledge. I looked over my shoulder into the drop. Being a good captain, I knew when to abandon ship. I shouted, "Jump!" and we both leaped for the rock. I scrambled up and made a dive for the canoe, but the bow slipped out of reach as the canoe went backward over the ledge.

Not surprisingly, the canoe navigated the rapid just fine without us. It cleared the ledge smoothly, bypassed the next two rocks, crossed the river, and parked itself gently on shore in a quiet eddy. Jim and I just sat on our rock, looking at each other. Just then we saw Donna and John starting down the rapid above us. They hadn't seen our little episode, so I waved them in to shore. As they came to a stop, they looked at us in confusion, wondering how we had parked our canoe a hundred meters downstream on the other side of the river, and then returned to sit on this rock to wait for them. We just smiled and began helping them with their canoe, amazed again at how easy it is to get into trouble.

EDITOR: *No matter how simple a decision seems to be, thoroughly evaluate it for risk. Gather all the necessary information—and by all means avoid complacency.*

A SITUATION ON THE KANANASKIS

Jim Buckingham

T WAS A WARM DAY ON THE KANANASKIS, a small river that tumbles through the front ranges of the Rocky Mountains just east of Banff National Park in Alberta. Six of us were paddling together in three canoes. The group was of mixed experience, and we were short experienced whitewater sternmen, so I convinced Louise to stern one of the canoes, which I knew she didn't really want to do. While she had many years of canoe-tripping experience on rivers and lakes, practically all of it had been in the bow. To make it easier for her—or so I thought—I gave her a canoe that she was familiar with, one she had sterned on many flatwater trips. This was a Brigden Model 20: originally designed to meet the specs of a certain long-distance flatwater race, it was really quite fun for short trips in small lakes. The canoe is very narrow, with a V-shaped hull and no rocker. These features make it easy to paddle swiftly in a straight line, but difficult to turn quickly in a tight situation.

Although not very experienced in canoes, Alice, Louise's paddling partner, was confident in all type of boats and strong, athletic, and cool in tough situations. I assured Louise that I knew the river well and that Mary and I would be in the lead at all times. The other two paddlers, John and Lorna, would bring up the rear. I planned to choose conservative lines, so all she had to do was follow me. This stretch of the Kananaskis was no more than class 2, a typical rocky, swift mountain river.

Everything went well through most of the trip. Louise had some difficulties maneuvering her canoe exactly where she wanted it to go, but there were no real problems. We were all having a fine day as we approached the bottom portion of the river, just a few turns upstream of the planned take-out. We came to a fairly tight corner, with most of the water rushing to the outside. For a couple hundred feet along the outside edge, there was a vertical rock wall twenty feet high.

Mary and I were in the lead, and I eddied out on the gravel beach at the inside of the bend. Louise, however, was unable to get the angle for the turn quickly enough. The powerful current swept her canoe to the outside, where it hit the cliff sideways, pinned against the rock by the force of the current. When practicing on flatwater, it's easy to say "If you broadside against an obstacle, lean downstream toward it" to keep from capsizing. But in reality it's quite difficult to get much of a downstream lean if your canoe is against a vertical cliff. What we didn't know is that this cliff had been severely undercut below the waterline. The current flowed undiminished under the lip of the rock, and the force on the bottom of the canoe was extreme.

It took only a moment for the upstream gunwale to sink. In a flash, the canoe was pushed under the overhang, upside down and pinned again. The women were now under it, trapped by the force of the current. Struggling in the darkness, Alice was able to pull herself toward the bow of the canoe, which was barely underwater. She managed to thrust her head above the surface just outside the overhang and immediately looked for Louise but could see no sign of her. Despite the current, she was able to work hand over hand along the gunwale, reaching under the water for Louise. The stern was much deeper in the water, though, and Alice could neither see nor feel any part of Louise.

Mary and I had already started across the river to help. It

took only a few seconds to rescue Alice from her tight spot and get her safely to shore. The canoe, however, was still pinned under the cliff, and we couldn't figure out how to get to it. Suddenly, after what seemed like forever, Louise popped up more than a hundred feet downstream. Mary and I immediately paddled like crazy in her direction. Louise was swept into another bit of rough water and went under again. She was under only an instant before Mary and I reached her and were able to pull her out.

Once Louise recovered somewhat, she told us that she had been pinned under the stern seat but was able to move slightly by pushing against the canoe. She quickly found that the only direction she could go was down. She made a powerful thrust with her legs and was swept clear of the canoe. The current then dragged her down and under the point of the overhang. Fortunately, the undercut—and the cliff—ended at that point, and she was pushed out into deep water. As she was carried swiftly downstream, it took her several more seconds to struggle to the surface.

With the excitement over, we sat down to eat lunch on top of the cliff. The Kananaskis is one of the few dam-controlled rivers in the Canadian Rockies, and while we were eating the power company reduced the flow. When we noticed the water level dropping, we looked for the canoe, only to find that the reduced current pressure had washed it clear of the cliff. We eventually found it two bends downstream, caught on a rock. There were twenty-one tears or punctures in the fiberglass.

This day was a perfect example of how, even on easy rivers, things can go very wrong very fast. We were lucky. Had any debris been trapped under the overhang, Louise probably would not have made it out. As trip leader, I was at fault for choosing a river that was unsuitable for the skills of *all* the participants. I let myself be carried away by the thought of what a fine piece of river this was to share with friends, rather than choosing water they were capable of handling.

EDITOR: *Both in the pretrip planning stage and once you're on the river, it's difficult to deal with a group of paddlers whose skills and abilities vary widely. As trip leader, by the time you realize that the level of difficulty on the water exceeds the ability of one of the paddlers, it may be too late.*

BROKEN YOKE GORGE ON THE WATHAMAN
Laurel Archer

E NEED TO MAKE OUR WAY river right," Sheila said. The speed of the boiling green water was increasing.

"OK," I replied, immediately picking a route through spray and boulders. Pry to avoid a pillow, draw to slip by another. My sister and I were reading and running technical class 3 water on the Wathaman River in northern Saskatchewan, and we were having a blast on our last day on this wilderness river. It had been over a week of granite gorges, long continuous rapids, and tough bushwhacking portages.

We were a finely tuned team. I was paddling bow and enjoying it immensely. This was my first chance to paddle tandem this summer, after paddling solo for thirty-five days in the northern wilderness. I couldn't have asked for a better partner. Sheila was the queen of whitewater in the stern of her green Old Town Tripper, *Alfecca*. I felt as if we could run everything on this trip, and for the most part we had.

We were approaching the narrowest section of Stuart Rapids, the longest (at 1,600 meters) and most difficult rapid on the challenging Wathaman. The gorge walls looked like converging lines, it's that steep. There was a drop of some kind in the middle, but all I could see below was a funnel of white waves. It looked as if we would have to scout from shore.

"I think we'll have to eddy out river right after that big boulder before that drop!" I yelled. Everything started to speed up. I

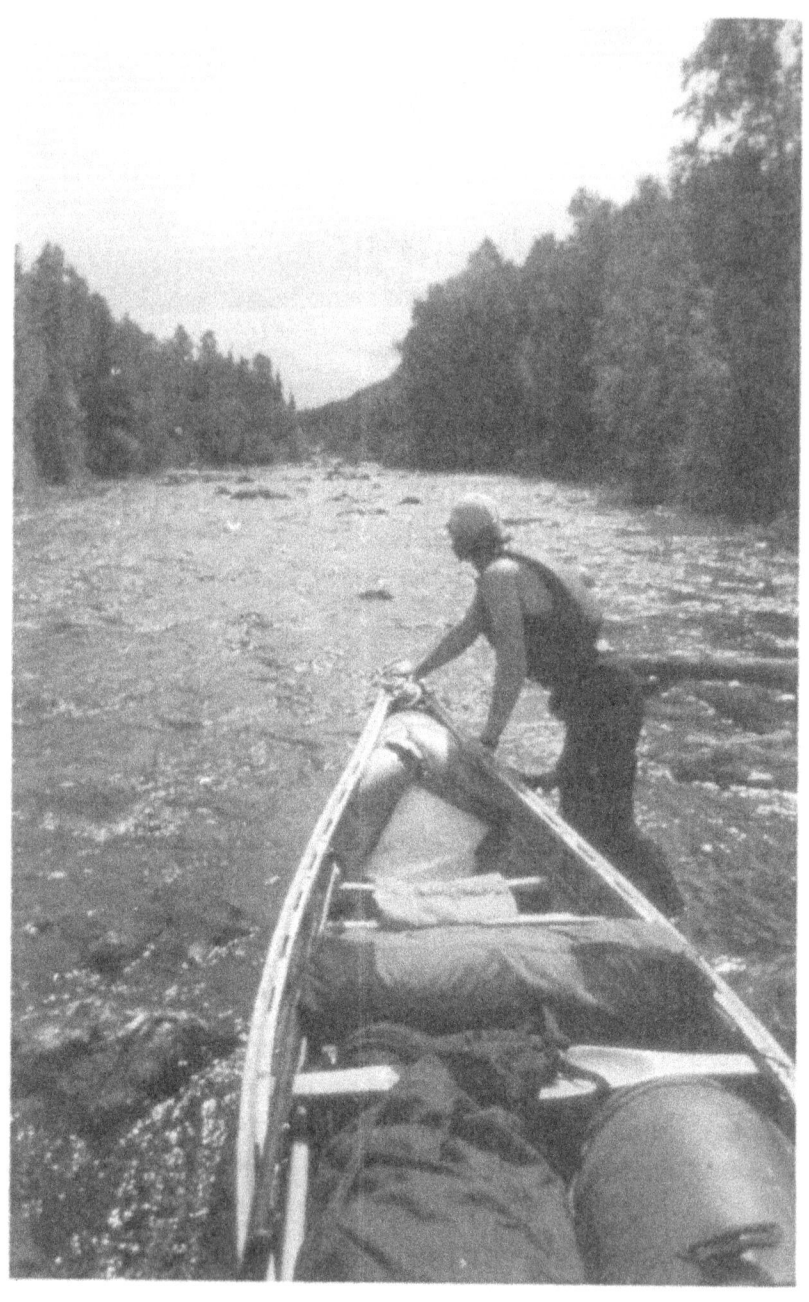

On the Wathaman River before the gorge.

strained to see farther. Was there a chute? A ledge? Could we just run it?

"River right after the boulder," Sheila confirmed the plan. We both struggled to maneuver around big rocks in the large waves.

We were just at the boulder, almost to the eddy, when I looked downriver again. We were almost on top of the big rapid in the narrowest part of the gorge.

"Definitely something happening there!" I exclaimed, and initiated the turn into the shore eddy. Then I peeked over my shoulder again—just one more look. The chute was too steep to run without filling up, but there was another smaller ledge on river right that might work. I turned back, expecting to be in the eddy.

Crack! The bow collided with a flat rock on shore. Stunned, I managed to jump out. I quickly crouched to examine the front of the canoe.

"Do we still have a bow?" asked Sheila.

"It's fine. There isn't anything I can see," I said with relief. "Wow. What was that sound?"

"I don't know. Weird. Let's tie up to one of those trees up there on the cliff and see what's with that drop down there."

Sheila turned to get the stern painter. "That's what that crack was." She pointed at the ash yoke: the wood was split along the grain, having snapped under the impact of the barrels coming forward at high velocity when we hit.

It took a minute to sink in: the boat was broken. We now had a fragile craft that would easily wrap, and a class 4 drop and two more long, difficult rapids to go before Wathaman Lake. I couldn't believe I hadn't done something, at least thrown in a pry to turn us a few centimeters before contact. Why did I have to look downstream one more time? Why did I want to keep going, pushing the limits of safety by not getting out of the boat to scout? For the rush. That was the truth, and now the consequences.

There was nothing to do but find a way to line the drop and attempt a repair at the end of Stuart Rapids. After a fingers-and-toes line across the face of a black, lichen-covered cliff, we got back into our banana boat. With a far less cavalier attitude, we navigated safely down to flatwater.

We improvised a thwart with a sturdy piece of birch and some lashing. Given a fold-up saw and some cord, Sheila's quite a carpenter in a pinch. As we saw to the repairs, I told her, "I feel like I could have prevented this, at least throwing in a pry to turn us a bit."

She looked up from her work, "I could have done something, too. Don't worry about it." It was unspoken, but we both knew we would be more conservative now.

As it turned out, the rest of day was full of interesting events, all outside our control: a huge electrical storm we had to wait out twice, a windstorm that pinned us on shore, and then finally a forest fire on the shore of the narrow lake opposite our floatplane pickup point.

To this day, however, it still rankles me that I had become too cocky. I got caught pushing it, anticipating the next rapid rather than dealing with the task at hand. It could have been worse, but a broken yoke is no joke in the middle of a Wathaman gorge.

EDITOR: *When you're very good at what you do, it's often hard to keep in mind that things can still go wrong. A moment of inattention is all it takes.*

THE ONE-MINUTE MEASUREMENT
John Silver

NE OF THE THINGS I LOOK AT when paddling is how to lead people to make good decisions about whether or not a set of rapids can be run successfully, given the parameters of the trip.

While on a trip from Labrador into Québec on the Moise River, our group had a new participant who at the time had not done an expedition of similar magnitude. Tim was a good athlete and quick to pick up new skills, but after ten days of tough portages, constant rain, and having to fix everything from yokes to packs to tents, he was ready to stand outside the tent, hold his VISA card over his head, and conjure a chopper that would drop from the sky and take him home.

One of the rafting "rules" that clicked for me on this trip is the one-minute rule, which refers to the time allowed to decide whether or not a stretch of whitewater can be run. That doesn't mean that the route, rescue sites, and camera sites are decided within a minute, just that the question "Can we do it?" has to be answered in that time. If you can't answer that question in a minute, then the likelihood is that you're really just using the additional time to talk yourself into something that is probably both foolish and dangerous. This decision is not based solely on skill or desire but on how your team feels, the time of the day, and whether or not your brain is crippled with testosterone.

One evening, Debby and I ran a simple drop—a short, small

rapid with little vertical drop—where we became sloppy and didn't communicate well. There was one more drop left before we would reach our camping spot at the end of the rapid. We each took more than a minute to evaluate what should have been a straightforward case, but we stuck to the one-minute rule and decided to walk around. We were in lousy moods: it was the end of a long day, we had a communication screw-up at the previous drop, and we were both tired and hungry. Walking around was the right move for us under the circumstances.

Later in the trip, Tim and Blake were paddling together when we hit the Railway Rapid, a wonderful drop that is the last of the big drops before the Moise enters the mouth of the St. Lawrence Seaway. Tim had had it when they arrived at the rapid. In fact, he was already having trouble at the rapid just before this one. Blake recognized this, so they decided to walk around the rapids, even though we had all been gearing up for this run all day—indeed for the entire trip. Blake and Tim didn't sulk, but rather accepted that their whitewater trip was over.

Putting aside their egos allowed the paddlers to do what was right for them—a key element in avoiding poor decisions. Blake supported Tim even though it meant not doing the rapids, and Tim was comfortable enough to say to Blake that he didn't feel up to doing the rapids.

The one-minute rule and the ability to say "no" to running drops without facing criticism made this a safe but fun canoe trip. I would like to say that these two aspects have meant that I have never had to swim. Of course, that would be a lie, but at least I swam in safe rapids!

ALL IN A DAY'S WORK

Doug McKown and Jim Buckingham

OUG: STANDING ON SHORE WATCHING the chaos underway downstream, I couldn't believe that a simple day of
instruction had developed into a circus of near disaster. This was
the first day of our four-day canoe course on the Bow River in
Banff National Park in Alberta. Teaching canoeing on mountain
rivers is always a challenge. There are no pool and drop rapids
here, some sections are faster, others slower—but it just keeps
flowing. Once a capsize occurs, it's easy for participants to become separated if things aren't strictly controlled. And the water
is always cold: on this first weekend in June the water level was
high and running a balmy eight degrees Celsius.

Things had been going well. I was leading the first of the two
groups as we approached the final rapid, and Jim was leading
the second. Red Earth is a long but not difficult rapid that curves
back and forth with lots of waves and a few rocks. The main
rapid is about five hundred meters long, but there is still a lot of
current farther down. This rapid always makes an exciting finish
to the first day of the paddling course, and we have been using it
for many years.

My group came down one canoe at a time through the first section of the rapid. We stopped in a large eddy to wait for the arrival of the second group. They had been getting organized as
we left, so although I couldn't see them from our position in the
eddy, I knew they wouldn't be long.

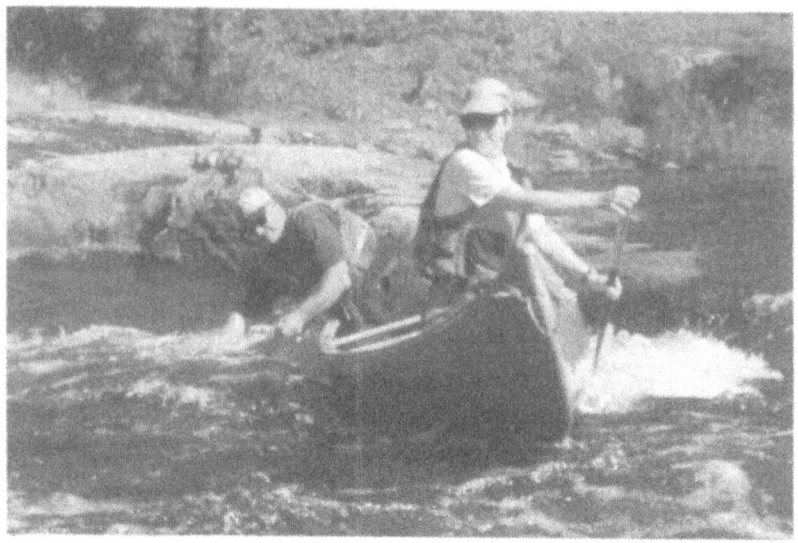

Jim and Donna performing a skills demonstration earlier in the day.

Jim: Doug's group had gone down the first section of the rapid while I was getting my group organized. On shore, I quickly explained what I expected the group to do. As I pulled out to make my demonstration run, I knew that Doug and his group would be on the beach just around the corner, although a curve in the river made it impossible for me to see that far. We usually gather both groups in that eddy, set up the safety boats, and then send the students down one canoe at a time.

My bowman, "Aaron," was an inexperienced student, but thousands of less experienced people have run this rapid without problem. And I had been paddling this section of river for more than twenty-five years. However, as I hit the first little waves at the top of the rapid, that was it. I have no idea what happened, but all at once we were swimming. I'm sure the rest of the class was as astonished as I was to see the instructor dump in such an easy spot. Doug was certainly surprised when the first glimpse he had of my group was my boat upside down and two people swimming alongside.

Doug: At first I couldn't tell what was happening. Then I realized that Jim and Aaron were floating by, waving at us. *This shouldn't have happened.* They were on the far side of the current, too far for a throw-bag rescue. No problem. I had two safety boats with me: Donna and a student ("Kim") in one, and Laura and Keith, two experienced paddlers, in the other. Just as Laura and Keith headed out to get Jim and Aaron, Aaron let go of the canoe. Now we had two separate rescues to make, so Donna and Kim headed out to get the swimmer.

I watched as they all headed down the rapid together. Just then I heard a shout upstream. Our third rescue canoe, with Brent and Mac aboard, was coming down the first part of the rapid to see what had happened to Jim. Brent and Mac were a little excited, and they capsized just as they turned toward my eddy. I was fast running out of safety boats. I jumped into my canoe solo and headed out to help them. I grabbed their canoe and did a quick T-rescue; they clambered back in as I steadied their boat. Once I thought they were under control, I pushed them off so I could get back to shore before the start of the next rapid. I was a little premature in my assessment, though. Brent and Mac were still getting organized as they headed into the rapid and promptly capsized again. Now I was in a quandary. If I went after them again, it would mean leaving the entire class, about ten canoes, on their own at the top of the rapid: not an acceptable option. I decided to leave Brent and Mac to their fate, since I knew there were still two safety boats somewhere downstream. I headed back to the beach, wondering how I was going to convince all the students that this was perfectly normal instructor behavior.

Now I was the only rescue/instructor canoe anywhere near the top of the rapid. Jim's group was still above us, still out of communication. I hoped they had been told to hang tight until they heard from us. No such luck. Just as I got to the beach, down came the first student canoe.

Meanwhile: Donna and Kim had connected with Aaron and towed him to shore at the bottom of the rapid. He was cold, but no worse for wear. Donna was about to get out and take care of him when she saw Brent and Mac swimming down the rapid with their canoe. Instructing Kim to stay where he was, she went to catch up with Brent and Mac and do another T-rescue. This time Brent and Mac were able to get to shore, and Mac started jogging back upstream to see if I needed help.

Keith and Laura had caught up to Jim and performed an excellent T-rescue. They steadied the canoe and he climbed in, but he was very cold and already beginning to lose coordination. He had climbed into the stern of the canoe, creating an unstable situation. Before he had a chance to get organized, his canoe hit a rock and he went down again. Keith and Laura went after him right away, performing another T-rescue as they all floated farther and farther downriver. Jim was getting seriously cold and hypothermic by this time. He had already been in the water for five or ten minutes and was having difficulty trying to get back into his canoe, capsizing yet again. That was the last I saw of them as they disappeared around a bend almost a kilometer downstream. I later learned that Keith and Laura were finally able to tow Jim and his canoe to shore. By that time Jim was unable to climb out of the water unassisted. He was confused and barely seemed aware of what was going on. However, after some quick care, dry warm clothes, and a warm drink he was alert—and completely embarrassed about the whole episode.

Back at the beach, I watched the students come down, hoping that nothing else would go wrong. All went well until the second to last student canoe capsized right in front of me. Luckily, I was able to use my throw bag to bring both students and the canoe safely into shore. With all the students together at last, things settled down. Eventually, we were able to get completely reorganized, finishing off the day without further incident.

EDITOR: *This day was a perfect example of how quickly things can go wrong and how quickly a simple situation can deteriorate. Although we had reviewed what to do if an instructor became a swimmer, not everyone completely understood or remembered the plan. Thankfully, no one was hurt and Jim's hypothermia wasn't serious, but it took much longer than it should have to get this situation under control. Communication and proper planning would have prevented the snowballing string of problems.*

NEVER GIVE UP

Cliff Jacobson

THE LOWER FIVE MILES OF THE MacFarlane River in northern Saskatchewan flow through a high-walled canyon punctuated by huge rapids and falls, with just enough clear routes to tease the imagination. Still, only a fool would run this canyon because, once you're committed, the only way out is downriver.

We put ashore at the head of the canyon on river right, climbed a high sandy hill, and then methodically began to scout the drop. For a while, we followed a well-used animal trail along the canyon rim that appeared to be the portage, but it ended in impenetrable vegetation after about a quarter mile. There was a huge rapid—and canoe-eating hole—just where the trail ended. A narrow ledge jutting from the canyon wall would make lining the rapid a tricky operation; if we missed our cue, there were more rapids and a falls below. We studied this obstacle for a long time before giving up and resuming our search for the elusive portage.

I assumed the portage must lie farther inland, so I set a compass course ninety degrees out from the river and hiked for fifteen minutes. Nothing but more thick bush. I returned to the head of the canyon and tried again. This time a friend and I walked due east for thirty minutes by compass and GPS. Again, a blank. Could the portage be on the other side of the river?

I studied the far shore through my binoculars. The bush looked thicker, the canyon wall steeper, and there was no easy take-out point. Perhaps there was a clear route on top, but ferrying across the three-hundred-yard-wide rapid-filled river wouldn't be easy. One screw-up and we'd be committed to the canyon.

Of course, we could wade our boats a few hundred yards upstream in waist-deep water and cross with a little more room. But the bushy left bank led us to believe we were already on the correct bank. Besides, the animal trail that followed the canyon rim began right where we had beached our canoes. Another reason for staying put was the ancient blaze we found nearby on a large spruce tree. We guessed that the mark, which must have been cut by an ax, was at least ten years old. The sun was dropping and we were weary of exploring, so we decided to pitch camp and search afresh the next morning.

Long experience in the Canadian bush has taught me that there is a way around every obstacle, and I have driven this point home repeatedly on my trips and in my books. But four additional hours of intensive searching had revealed nothing, and there was hushed talk of running or lining the canyon.

We were exhausted and out of ideas when a friend said an animal trail that began at the water's edge continued into the woods and "headed in the right direction but disappeared after a hundred yards."

"Would you look at it again with me?" I asked.

"Sure."

We had found the portage, though it hadn't been used in many years. A maze of wrist-thick trees blocked the route, and getting canoes through, let alone packs, would be impossible without some work.

We rounded up our cutting tools—one three-quarter-length ax, one large hatchet, one full-frame saw, and one jackknife—and went to work. Two days later we had opened the old canyon trail and portaged everything across.

There is always a safe way around every obstacle on a canoe trip, and you will find it if you slow down and keep a clear head.

Only in the most dire circumstances would I cut live trees on a canoe trip, but trails grow over quickly on little-used routes, and government agencies don't have the money or staff to keep them clear, particularly in remote areas. I don't know what we would have done without our axes and saws.

It may be politically correct to leave your ax and full-frame folding saw at home on a canoe trip, but it may also be a bad idea if you're tripping off the beaten path and have to clear a portage.

MISHAP ON THE NOTAKWANON RIVER
Bob Henderson and Warren Trimble

UMPING A FULLY LOADED CANOE and taking an un-
scheduled swim in a remote northern river adds up to a serious affair. No paddler likes to make foolish mistakes—never
mind many mistakes in succession—on such a trip. Admitting our
mistakes is harder still. By drawing on our field notes we hope
to offer as authentic a review of events as possible.

First, the setting. We had flown in near the headwaters of the
Notakwanon River on the Québec side of the height of land
marking the Québec–Labrador border. We had four days of shallows and lakes ahead of us before accessing the river corridor
itself. Our group was made up of four paddlers who were comfortable running whitewater, in two canoes: a Kevlar seventeen-
footer and a big-volume ABS canoe. The two of us were in one
canoe, and David and Steve in the other. The Upper Notakwanon
River is a long way from anywhere; the nearest settlement on
the coast was about two weeks or more from our starting point.
Wanting time to hike, we had given ourselves sixteen days to
reach Davis Inlet on the Labrador coast.

Warren: Today we enter the river from the headwater lakes. I'm
a bit anxious, but satisfied with our pretrip preparation and the
time we've had as a group and all else. Would like another boat,
though. Three canoes and six people are safer for a river like this.
The distant view of the river valley (which we are now so *close* to
being in) was incredible all day. At times we looked above the hills.

We passed a rock buttress that we had watched much of the day. The day was a succession of rapids (each requiring a line or shoot decision), outflow bay; rapids, outflow bay; and so on for fifteen kilometers or so. We did well, both canoes reading the water, picking routes, making good decisions. Late in the day we faced one more long (two kilometers) stretch of whitewater to line or run; it led directly to a falls, where we planned to camp. After scouting the first three-hundred-meter section, we decided we could run that piece, then read the rest as we traversed an intervening stretch of flatter water.

We come to our appropriate "out," but instead of lining the rest we arrogantly stay "in" the current. Probably our egos are doing our thinking for us. We make for the middle and indeed the water is readable, though faster than we imagined. Bob and I, in the lead canoe for the moment, find ourselves too much toward the middle, too far downstream without scouting, rounding a broad corner without knowledge of flow, and as luck would have it, facing a ledge. We swamp! Bob grabs the wanigan and camera box (which pops up to him), while I turn and grab two day-packs and one big pack as the canoe disappears under us.

Bob: The canoe didn't have a sprayskirt on or packs tied in yet because we haven't reached the falls, the place after which we figured we would need to get set up for running (?) or long-lining whitewater. (Sheepishly, we admit to reading the map more than the river.) We kick to shore with what gear we can handle in little time, it seems, though with no eddies the arrival is difficult.

Warren: Bob makes shore upstream of me, and I see him running the shore, presumably looking for the canoe and a big pack we can't afford to lose.

Bob: I can't see either of them.

Warren: At this point, Dave and Steve, who are following us, see the results and likewise commit to the ledge, with no other real option. With their bigger boat and bow sprayskirt, they take in water but punch through and arrive close to Bob.

Bob: We have little dialogue. Just get out, get gear, and look for the canoe. We then run downstream to look for stuff, never seeing the canoe! Warren is following the pack. A guitar in a bright yellow stuff sack floats high and easy to see. Warren wades out into the current for the pack but misses when the pack changes direction. I do this once as well, but the pack moves on. Eventually, after chasing it three to five hundred meters, we lose sight of the pack and, discouraged, wait for the guitar in its stuff sack, which floats gracefully into the only calm pool in this two-kilometer stretch above the falls. Guitar saved. Later we will discover it's OK and still in tune.

Warren: As we begin to walk back upstream, I see the pack bobbing across the river in an eddy, but we can't get to it. Giving that up for the moment, we rush back to check on the canoe. What we see is odd: the canoe is high in the water, right side up, half-filled, and bobbing in the current (not out in the middle, but not close either—about twenty meters out). It has been snagged on its fifteen-meter lining rope, which must have looped or knotted or bunched on the bottom. It seems fixed permanently. Strange for a floating rope! We decide on our options:

1. A tethered swimmer struggles to the canoe and both are towed back. If the current is too strong to release the rope that is jammed to the riverbed, the swimmer hooks himself to the boat and cuts the line (trying to save as much of it as possible, of course—as if that were possible).

2. Three of us pile into the other canoe and use an upstream ferry to approach the boat, with the third member fixing a line to ferry it back. But this option puts our remaining boat at risk.

Bob: I volunteer for option 1. Warren's reply is, "You're married and have kids. Dave and Steve aren't the cause of all this. So, realistically, it should be me." OK. Warren puts on two life jackets and a farmer John wet suit retrieved from a pack. We tie double fisherman's knots to make a tow rope of thirty meters. Fortunately, we have carabiners and know how to rig a harness system.

Warren: We are set for the canoe rescue, but as I walk away up-

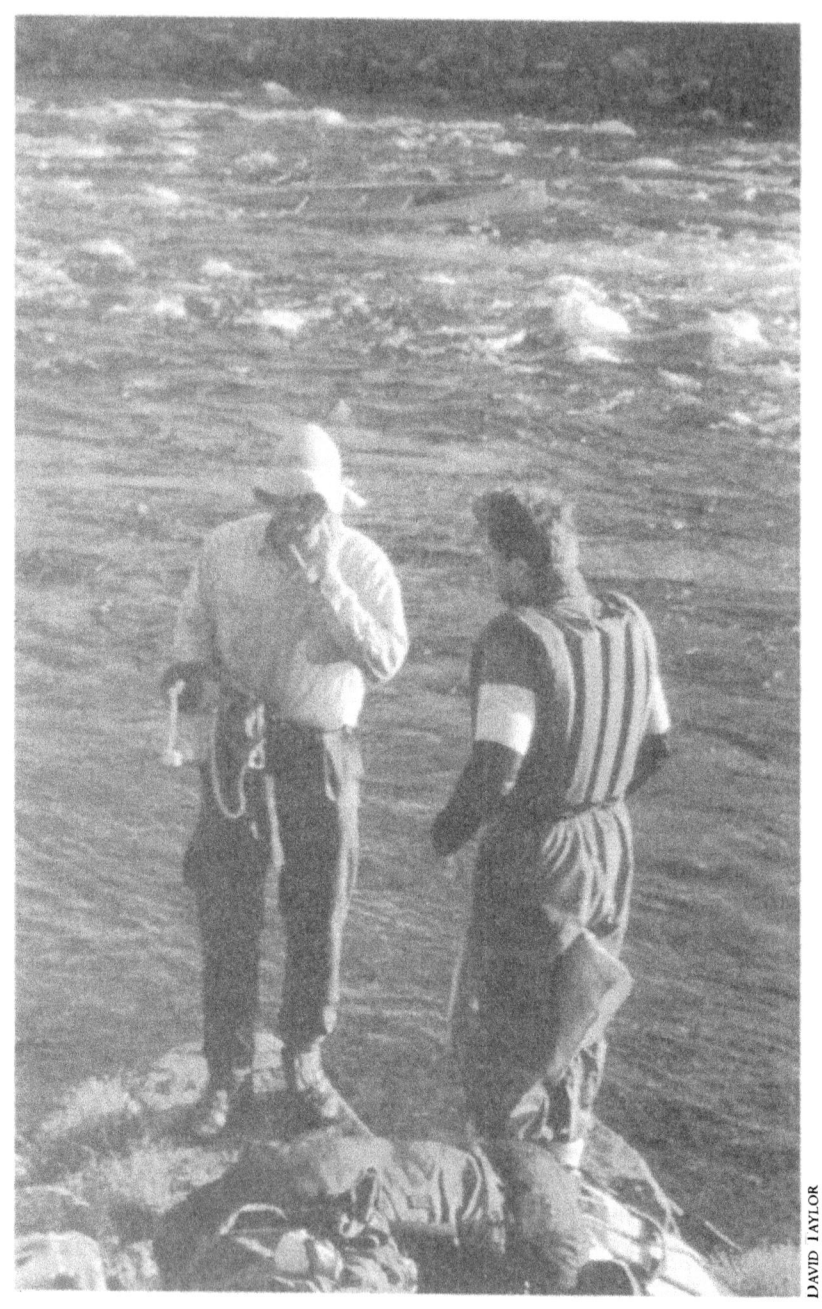

Warren and Bob prepare to rescue the canoe.

UP THE CREEK

stream, preparing to jump in, I'm told to stop. I look back to see that we are tied in wrongly, and I'm not attached to the line they're going to pull on. The comic overtones of the situation relieve some of our anxiety. Then, checking the rope as I head upstream, we acknowledge without speaking that we're all apprehensive, that we all understand the gravity of the situation, that we all trust one another, and that we'll do what is necessary. This, along with Dave's perception check, takes the edge off my tremendous fear. I have been viewing this as a one-shot, life-or-death attempt to retrieve a canoe, without which we are in deep trouble, but then Dave says, "It's getting late, and we have to make our first attempt. Then we'll know what changes to make for the next attempt." He has no idea how powerfully reassuring this is for me. Still, at first, I can't bring myself to jump in. After a brief gut check of contemplation and meditation, I plunge. I reach the boat on my first attempt and clip the carabiner onto the boat. They seem to pull with all their energy while I yell with fear, "Pull pull pull!" I'm hitting rocks with my body (I can't seem to get into the safety position). Bob runs into the water to help me up. Exhilarated, teary-eyed, I think of death, trust, and love.

Bob: The canoe damage is minor: an inner gunwale busted through its middle three to five feet, the bow and stern deck tips busted off, and a bad crease in the Kevlar. We load our gear (which Dave and Steve have carried here from the site of our swamping) in the two canoes and line them down the rapids to a possible campsite three hundred meters downstream—close enough to the twenty-two-meter falls to give us the willies if we care to think about it, which we don't. Warren and I then line the ABS boat farther down to where we last saw the pack. It's still there, as expected, and we retrieve it with an upstream ferry over and back. When we make it back to the campsite the tent is up and dinner is on.

We were lucky. The boat was weakened but repairable. We lost a map and the poles for one of our tents, but there was little food damage. We could cram three in one tent and use the poleless tent as a semipoled bivvy sack. We had made a mistake with possible dire consequences, but we had sorted it out. If we had lost that canoe, two of us would have had to stay right there seeking open ground for an air rescue while the other two paddled to our planned destination at Davis Inlet. The falls, too, was too close for comfort. These scenarios lurked in our minds while we worked through our rescue efforts, but fortunately there was little time to dwell on such matters.

When a mishap (OK, a stupid chain of mistakes) suddenly happens (OK, is precipitated by human error) there is perhaps an astonishing realization: "Hey, this is my hobby, my holiday, my recreation. How did events bring me to the real possibility of sitting out on the Labrador plateau, with or without gear, waiting for an air rescue? How did events bring us to a point where we are sending a swimmer into a northern river?" Yes, dumping a fully loaded canoe in a remote northern river is a serious affair.

In the early 1930s, not far south from our Notakwanon location, traveler Elliott Merrick mused (and later recorded in his classic book, *True North*): "To find oneself in the interior of Labrador . . . without a canoe would be almost synonymous with finding oneself dead."

Now, we suddenly found ourselves taking comfort from overhead NATO jet contrails. That is no way to explore the canoe heritage of Labrador. Happily, our "mishap" remained just that. We were in the interior of Labrador with one beat-up canoe, one crippled tent, and without maps for a few days, but it could have been worse.

EDITOR: *Even experienced paddlers can misplace their safety awareness at times. I believe this has less to do with conceit than simple complacency. No matter how experienced you are, think through every action and assess all consequences. It sounds so obvious. So why is it the hardest thing to do?*

KEYSTONE CANOEISTS
Doug McKown

IM, MARY, DONNA, AND I had decided to make a trip down the Foster River, a picturesque waterway running through the Shield country just north of the Churchill River. It had been a hot, dry summer in Saskatchewan, which meant that we would be able to run many rapids that might demand portaging at higher water levels. It also meant that we would be lining many rapids that normally could be paddled. We encountered one of these rapids in the middle of a hot, calm afternoon.

After running a small rapid to a calm pool, Jim and I hiked down the rocky shore to see what lay ahead. It was a long, boulder-filled rapid, and a capsize here, so close to the start, could mean trouble. While the Foster is a small river where drowning was unlikely, we didn't like the possibility of damaging one of only two canoes in the wilderness of northern Saskatchewan.

We successfully lined my canoe over the two ledges at the start of the rapid—one person positioning the canoe and one holding the upstream line. If possible, we always line with one rope to avoid the hazards of failed communication and coordination. Back at the top, we secured the lining rope to the bow loop of Jim's canoe. Jim held the rope while I positioned the canoe and prepared to send it on its way. When Jim signaled he was ready, I gently pushed the canoe out into the current, aiming for the center of the first ledge. Gliding around a rock, the canoe slid gracefully over the ledge in perfect position, dropping into the foaming pool below. I called to Jim to hold firm on the lining rope to pull the canoe back to shore. He braced himself and held firm, but the knot in the lining rope came untied, and the canoe headed down the rest of rapid on its own.

After a moment of frozen surprise, panic ensued. As this was Jim's canoe, he hopped downstream from rock to rock, trying to reach my canoe in time to rescue his. With only moments to spare, he leaped into my canoe with Donna, and they paddled furiously in a valiant attempt to catch his wayward canoe. However, in the excitement of the moment, Jim failed to notice that the canoe was securely tied to a large, solid tree. They quickly came to an abrupt, frustrating stop. I almost fell off my rock with laughter: Keystone canoeists strike again!

Luckily, Jim's canoe negotiated the next big ledge and a major portion of the following rapid just fine on its own. It came to rest quietly in an eddy at the river's edge.

As we reorganized and headed downstream, I pondered how fast a lining situation can go wrong. This shouldn't happen. You should have excellent control over all factors when you choose to line your canoe; yet lining continues to cause many dangerous situations for river paddlers. While this incident was harmless, it is never safe to become complacent about lining.

EDITOR: *Losing or breaking equipment in the wilderness is no laughing matter. Lining requires careful planning, continuous communication, and attention to detail—and having an alternate plan doesn't hurt, either.*

COOL ON THE CREDIT RIVER

Toni Harting

TUPID? OF COURSE IT WAS STUPID! Incredibly so. In hindsight, it's beyond me why I ever decided to run that little chute in the broken dam across the Credit River.

We were making every mistake in the book: tackling whitewater in a canoe that was too short, too wide, and keeled; we weren't scouting from shore; and we had no waterproof pack with extra clothing, no waterproof camera case, and no protec-

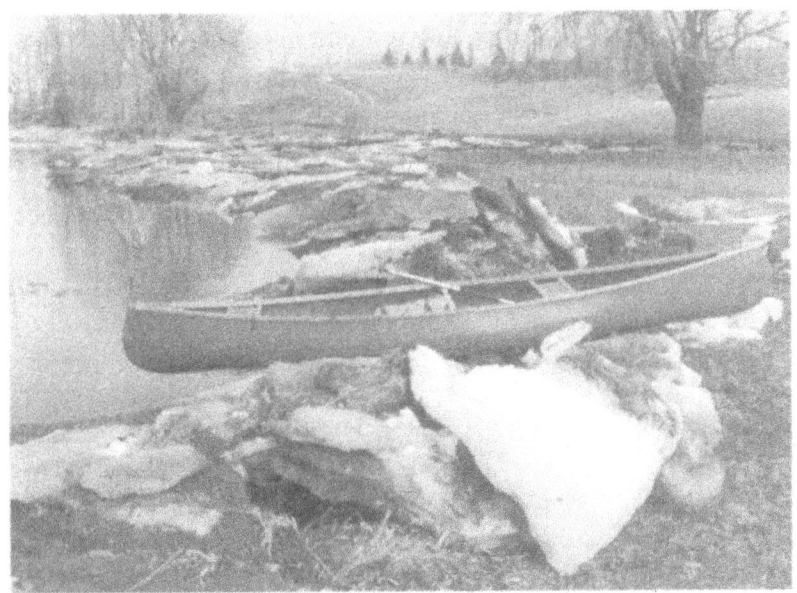

Putting in on the Credit River.

tive dry suits in case we fell into the freezing water. In fact, we had made no appropriate preparations at all for a cold-water trip in March.

It all happened so fast, I just couldn't believe it. Ria and I were drifting slowly toward the fifty-centimeter drop, a little too far left as we neared the edge. Then the bow went down. We hit the wave on the left at the wrong angle and at the wrong point, and in the blink of an eye were swimming and gasping for air in the icy water. Everybody swamps a canoe now and then: it's all part of the sport. But not in March, a few days after break-up, in a river with its banks still covered with huge blocks of ice.

Except for my damaged pride and a waterlogged camera, we came off pretty well. Mostly thanks to sunny, windless weather and a supportive group of Wilderness Canoe Association members. They got us out quickly, helped us dry off, and gave us warm clothing. We escaped hypothermia this time, but if we'd been alone on this trip, it would have meant big trouble.

A lesson learned the hard way is a lesson not easily forgotten. Next time we'll do it right so we don't needlessly endanger ourselves and spoil the trip for the rest of the party. I'll make the correct preparations and the right on-stream decisions, and above all, I'll leave the know-it-all confidence of the experienced old-timer at home. After all, it's never too late to learn.

A TRAGEDY ON THE BOW

Doug McKown

IT WAS SUPPOSED TO BE A SIMPLE TRIP. Two experienced canoeists were guiding a group of novice paddlers on an
overnight trip on the Bow River in Alberta. This section of the
Bow, in the front ranges of the Rocky Mountains, is very pleasant: the river is relatively shallow, with moderate currents, few
rocks, and no rapids. The main difficulty is choosing the proper
route, as the river braids extensively. The hazards of the route
include very cold waters and sweepers and logjams, which are
found along the shores and around islands. However, the moderate current and low shorelines mitigate these hazards, making it
safe for novice paddlers.

The two guides, John and Laura, were leading ten novices,
with a total of six canoes on the trip. As with most group trips,
organization and travel time took a toll, and the group didn't get
onto the river until 2:15 p.m. With Laura in the lead canoe and
John in the last canoe, the group headed downstream.

The beginners were having the usual problems. However, with
continuous instruction and practice, they were mostly able to
keep their canoes going straight, and to get to shore as necessary. Although the group spread out from time to time, everyone
was improving, and everyone was having a good time. There
were regular stops in eddies to collect the canoes and make sure
everyone was under control.

As the river became more braided, route finding became more

of a priority. Once again, Laura stopped the group in an eddy to ensure that all the paddlers were OK. Somehow the canoes became a little spread out, though, and during the reorganization John became the lead canoe. Prepared to continue downriver, John was faced with a choice of four river channels, three of which had visible logjams and sweepers.

The fourth channel appeared to be clear, at least as far as he could see. Although John had not been down that particular channel in the past, the current was only moderate and it seemed easy enough. By the time the group was committed to the channel, John could see that it was split again around a small island. The main channel on the left was completely blocked by a large sweeper and logjam. The only exit was a small channel that branched off to the right, directly opposite the logjam.

John immediately headed for the right shore and the slow water of the small exit channel. He landed on the inside of the corner, across from the logjam. Signaling to the oncoming canoes, John got the next two boats safely into shore. The fourth canoe was not so lucky. The paddlers were unable to get completely out of the main current in time, and instead of making it to the exit channel, their canoe became stuck on the edge of the logjam. Mary and Joanne in the fifth canoe were having similar trouble. They were coming down the channel entirely in the main current. Able to do no more than turn their canoe sideways, they floated broadside directly into the logjam.

As Laura rounded the curve above, she saw both canoes stuck on the logjam. Immediately identifying this as a critical situation, she quickly made her way to the right bank. John and Laura shouted instructions, but Mary and Joanne couldn't maintain their balance. The current flipped the canoe upstream, throwing both into the freezing water. Mary and Joanne were pushed beneath the boat and disappeared under the logjam.

John and Laura charged across the river, frantically searching for some sign of them. Mary surfaced in the middle of the logjam, stuck in some logs but breathing, with her head above water. The students managed to get her out of the water and to safety. There was still no sign of Joanne.

Then they spotted her, trapped in the branches about a meter below the surface. John jumped into the water but in the freezing water was unable to free her. A knife was brought from shore, and John cut Joanne's life jacket and clothing free from the branches. It probably took about seven minutes to get her head above water, but she was still tangled in the branches. John performed artificial respiration for the next ten minutes while the rest of the group worked to pull Joanne up onto the logjam, where CPR could be performed.

During this time, Laura had made sure the rest of the group was safe and under control, then took one of the canoes to get help. They weren't far from the highway, but it was still two hours before rescue workers could actually reach Joanne. They continued to work on her while evacuating her to the local hospital, but it was too late. She was pronounced dead at the hospital.

EDITOR: *Even the simplest situations can prove deadly. What seemed like a small misjudgment in route finding actually involved many related decisions about the students' level of ability and understanding, the probability of meeting such a hazard on a relatively "safe" section of river, how far downriver should be scouted, the amount of time and space the students needed to get to shore, and what options there were for reaching a canoe in trouble.*

A BAD CHOICE ON THE MANIGATOGAN

Dean McLeod

GROUP OF YOUNG ADULTS were enjoying a postgraduation canoe trip down the Manigatogan River in Manitoba. Recent rains had resulted in high water levels, even for mid-June, but the weather had been beautiful and the water was reasonably warm. Bob and his partner had taken the least experienced paddler as a third in their canoe. One of the other two canoes also had three paddlers, and the remaining canoe had just two.

The trip leader, Bob, was bone weary after a strenuous day of dealing with the pushy, deadly force of the high water. Late in the day, at the end of a lengthy portage around a class 5 chute, the trail sloped steeply down a ridge of bedrock for sixty meters, ending in flooded willows and a fast, rough eddy. The water below the chute was bursting downstream, causing the level at the put-in eddy to surge from ankle deep to up over the knee and down again like a constant boiling cauldron.

Bob knew there was a safer, easier put-in a hundred meters downstream. However, changing plans at this point would have required moving tired people, canoes, and heavy gear back up the rocky ridge, followed by scouting, bushwhacking, and swatting bugs to put in through thick, flooded willows. Bob decided to go ahead with the launch, even though many group members had strong misgivings. He stood knee to waist deep in the roiling water of the eddy, holding each canoe in turn while the paddlers prepared themselves. The first boat was put in and loaded with gear and its three occupants. The plan was for each canoe to sprint downstream against the eddy's current, holding a course close to the willows until passing out of the boils and waves.

The first canoe, which contained moderately experienced paddlers, took on a bit of water in the tailrace but stayed the course successfully, thanks to a mighty first push from Bob. While seeing the first group make it safely down bolstered Bob's confidence and quelled the others' concerns, it created an unreasonable expectation for the less experienced group that followed.

Bob had noticed how far downstream that first canoe had been swept; well out of communication range and too far to be an effective rescue boat if either of the next two canoes ran into difficulty. He also realized that if his canoe was the only rescue boat available, then the remaining duffer (third occupant) should not be with him. So he decided that the second canoe would carry three paddlers, despite their inexperience. The paddlers prepared as the first canoe had, but with less confidence and less skill to draw upon. Bob pushed them off, watching for a few seconds to see that his effort had headed them in the right direction before quickly wading back to shore to help his partner load and launch the last canoe. He knew that third boat needed to be launched quickly to help the second canoe if it had trouble.

The second canoe had inadvertently launched on the back of a surge wave, which robbed them of their initial momentum. They were turned toward the willows by the eddy current, and their reaction was slowed by the significant difference in weight due to the extra person. They were carried back to their launch point and were now accelerating backward, being drawn toward the huge standing waves at the outlet of the chute. Realizing their predicament, all three paddled as hard as they could. As two paddlers dug in with a vengeance on the same side, the third was recovering his paddle. Coordination failed, balance was lost, and the paddlers were thrown into the swirling waters as the canoe capsized.

The powerful currents prevented them from getting on their feet, and by the time Bob responded, jumping out as far as he dared, the canoe with the paddlers hanging on was well out of reach. The surging eddy swept the upstream end of the canoe until it was almost touching the main tongue of water racing out of the chute. When the canoe hit the main current seconds later, it had built up significant upstream speed. The loaded, water-filled canoe—along with the three swimmers still holding on—was spun dramatically into the current. Amid the confusion of waves, they were swirled and deposited right back in the eddy. Amazingly, all three swimmers had managed to hold onto the canoe.

They continued to hold on as the canoe began to accelerate upstream once again. However, Bob's paddling partner was now in position to launch her throw bag. It bounced off Bob's shoulder, continued through the air, and landed directly on top of the submerged canoe. Two of the swimmers grabbed the rope, holding tight while the canoe swung upstream and stuck against some bushes, held there by the eddy current.

From there, Bob was able to help all three wet, tired, and scared paddlers back to shore. One fishing rod was lost, but the rest of the gear was collected among the willows. With a little less respect for their leader's decision-making ability, five humbled, weary paddlers lugged their gear and boats through the willows to that safer put-in.

EDITOR: *Stress and fatigue can erode your ability to stay focused, evaluate the situation, and make a more difficult but correct choice.*

WHERE IS EVERYONE?

Bill Hosford

W HILE BECOMING SEPARATED on a canoe trip may not seem like a common problem, it's surprisingly easy to do, particularly on bigger rivers and large, island-filled lakes. The loss of contact between canoes can have serious consequences. Cooking equipment, tents, food, and other gear are probably not evenly distributed among boats, so some could end up without shelter or warm food if forced to go it alone.

One of the worst aspects of losing contact is that you may not know if the rest of your party is ahead or behind. If you are behind but don't realize it, waiting for the other canoes of course exacerbates the problem; if you are ahead, going faster will also just put more distance between you.

I have been in this situation on two occasions. The first took place on the Rupert River in Québec. There were two canoes in our party. After taking a break with the other boat, my partner and I paddled ahead and then stopped to answer the call of nature. As we approached shore, I asked my partner to look back to see if the other canoe was behind us. He couldn't see them, so when we finished our break, we waited for them to catch up. After a long wait, we decided to paddle upstream to see if they were in trouble. After a hard slog against the current, we reached our last contact point. Only then did we realize that they must have passed us while we were on shore.

We eventually did catch up to the other canoe, luckily before nightfall. They had seen us pulling in to shore and shouted to let us know where they were, but we hadn't noticed them.

The second time something similar happened was on the lower Nahanni River. In a solo canoe, my daughter had pulled into an eddy to photograph us as we paddled by. Although she shouted to alert us to her position, we neither heard nor saw her. Thinking she was still in front of us, we paddled faster to catch up. Eventually, we stopped to take stock of the situation, as we hadn't seen her for quite a while and were getting worried. While we were talking, she came into view upstream, paddling furiously. She was one angry paddler, thinking she had been left behind.

We were lucky, but these situations could have had serious consequences. There is no substitute for clear communication within a group.

EDITOR: *Evaluating a situation and making good decisions depends on communication. Without it, you quickly lose the ability to control events.*

HAVE MAP, WILL TRAVEL
John Buchanan

HE WEATHER FORECAST was for a nice weekend, so I phoned my usual canoeing companions, Sharon, Dave, and Ray, and we quickly planned a canoe trip to one of our favorite areas in the Canadian Shield. I threw some porridge and pasta into my pack along with a tent and sleeping bag, and met the others at dawn on Saturday morning. Because of the rush, we forgot a few things, although nothing important except a map. We had a black-and-white strip map showing our route, but no information on the adjacent areas. However, we had all been to Davidson Lake many times, and we reached our campsite that night with no difficulty.

The weather was even better than predicted: clear skies, calm breezes, and moderate temperatures. We were in no hurry to head home on Sunday, but neither are we the types to laze around camp. We decided to try another, longer route back that was only slightly off the map. We knew the general area and were certain that we could navigate a few kilometers without maps. We would be like the first fur traders, we told ourselves confidently.

The first portage was about half a kilometer to a tiny circular lake at the edge of the strip map. And that's where the trouble started. An extensive blowdown covered the portage trail, forcing us to detour through heavy brush. We quickly became lost but kept going in the general direction of the lake, believing we couldn't miss it. We eventually reached a lake, although it looked nothing like the small circular lake on the edge of the strip map. Tired of carrying the canoes, we put in and paddled around the lake. Ray quickly spotted a portage, and within a couple of hours we were back in familiar territory and on our way home.

That night I got out the topo map to try to figure out where we had been. On a full-color map, the circular lake we were searching for turned out to be a contour line.

For many years, during the second week of September Jack and I would paddle from Bird Lake to Bissett, Manitoba, via Woodland Caribou Provincial Park. We prided ourselves on taking a different route each year through the park's many lakes and interconnected waterways.

One year we planned to paddle up Royd Creek, cross a height of land, and drop into the Bloodvein River, a route that looked straightforward on the map. The first few days were uneventful, and by the third night we were camped at the end of an established portage trail.

The following morning we set out to blaze a trail to the next lake. Following a compass course, we began to cut a trail. It seemed to take much longer than anticipated, but eventually we arrived at the lake. After a refreshing drink we returned for the canoe and packs and were soon ready to explore new territory.

The lake didn't seem to match the map, but we felt we would quickly get our bearings once we got out of the small cove. We paddled out and were dumbfounded to find last night's campsite on the other side of the bay. We had spent the entire morning portaging back into the same lake we had started from!

We returned to our campsite and this time found the correct lake by dead reckoning.

Several years later Jack and I took a course on navigation. The instructor mentioned that the presence of iron ore, which is especially common in the Canadian Shield, can throw off compass readings, causing the user to wander about in circles around an ore body. Jack shot me a knowing look.

A few years ago I set out to paddle the Berens River, which flows into Lake Winnipeg in Manitoba, with Ryan and our usual companions, Gerry and Maureen. The Berens was running high that summer, with longer, more difficult rapids than usual. On several occasions we were so close to the shore that we were paddling in the trees on the flooded banks.

In addition to topo maps, we carried Real Berard's map of the river, which described the rapids, portages, sights, and history. For the first several days, the maps were accurate and informative, and with the strong current we were making excellent time downriver. However, we ultimately learned to regret our reliance on maps instead of our senses.

When we came to a rapid where the river doubled back on itself, we paddled as far downstream as possible before landing to scout. It was a short walk across the flat, narrow end of the peninsula. The rapid looked ferocious, at least a class 3 with several monstrous standing waves at the end. According to the map, the portage was located on river left—the opposite shore. The banks there looked steep and rough, but we decided to investigate.

We ferried the canoes across and crept along shore, looking for signs of a portage. About halfway down the rapid we entered a small backwater. To proceed farther downriver would have almost certainly resulted in a capsize, ferrying across looked risky and wouldn't improve our situation, and returning upriver was out of the question. The only option appeared to be straight up the bank. The only problem was the ten-foot cliff looming above our position.

Ryan, the tallest member of the group, managed to find enough handholds to pull himself—with an enthusiastic boost from the remaining canoeists—over the rim of the cliff. I threw him the front painter, and he hoisted all the packs to safety. Once Gerry and Maureen were also to the top, we pulled the canoes up, and I scrambled up behind them. We were finally together on top of the cliff with all our gear, but our troubles weren't over.

We found ourselves in an old burn populated by six-foot-tall spruce trees so densely packed that we had to cut our way through. It was several hours before we made it back to the river below the rapid. The portage, of course, was on river right at the wide end of the peninsula, just where logic dictated.

EDITOR: *Getting lost can be frightening and dangerous. Pretrip planning should help you avoid this, but when it does happen, even experienced paddlers may ignore the realities of the situation. You "bend the map," or try to make the map fit your surroundings or your surroundings fit the map. The longer you wait before making a logical, thorough evaluation of your situation, the worse the predicament may get.*

A BREAK AT THE END OF THE DAY
John Silver

HILE ON A TRIP DOWN THE PIGEON RIVER, on the busy and beautiful east side of Manitoba's Lake Winnipeg, I had the pleasure of spending time with several close friends of mine, Tim, Blake, and Al. At the end of a day of rapids, sunshine, horseflies, and the usual hysterical stories from Al, I was ready for a relaxing swim. We set up camp and I donned my life jacket and slipped into the water. It was just the right temperature, and I made sure that I stayed river right, where the small riffle felt more like a Jacuzzi tub than a rapid.

However, I broke one of the cardinal rules. I was tired and allowed myself to become complacent. While in the small, safe rapid, I allowed my body to relax and circulate around the eddy and then enter into the eddy on the main rapid. I noticed too late that I had crossed the eddy line and was now well into the rapid that took up most of the river channel. It was an ugly, circulating rapid with a good hole that sucked down anything close to the curl at the base of the rock wall. I floated helplessly as I was pulled up to the hole, sucked down, and then spit out—but not far enough to clear the grip of the recirculating current. I was carried back into the rapid again, but by this time my shouting had informed the group of my trouble. Al grabbed one of the throw bags and made a perfect toss, but I was unable to grab it. I was sucked back into the hole, but having survived round one, this time I was more aware of my surroundings.

The water tumbled me down and brought me back up, only to recirculate again. But this time I had figured out what I had to do. Harry Stimson, an experienced Manitoba paddler, used to tell people in this situation to "swim to the bottom to live," which is what I did this time: when the hole sucked me down the third time, I swam as hard as I could toward the bottom of the river. The current along the bottom of the river carried me clear of the recirculating water above, and I came to the surface well beyond the hole. I finally drifted to shore, where my group was waiting.

With good attention from the group members to make sure I was warmed, rehydrated, and fed, I recovered quickly, and we were able to continue on our way, but it could have been disastrous for the group—and for my family.

EDITOR: *Complacency strikes again. Communication and early intervention can often prevent a bad situation from getting worse, but pretrip planning and knowledge—in this case, John's understanding of the hydraulic action of the hole—may also help paddlers extricate themselves from a difficult situation.*

WHERE EXACTLY ARE WE?

Doug McKown

T WAS A BEAUTIFUL DAY to start a two-week canoe trip in northern Saskatchewan. Don and Bill were loading the final canoe into the twin Otter, while I took a few last photos. In no time, we were heading north over the vast green carpet of the Canadian Shield toward lower Foster Lake, the headwaters of the Foster River.

We could see an endless panorama of sparkling lakes joined by tiny ribbons of glistening water. We were mesmerized by the continuous grandeur for the entire forty-five-minute flight. Bill was taking pictures while I was talking to Donna, who was a little green around the gills, when we felt the plane begin to descend. A quick circle and then the pilot took us down on the wide, calm lake.

When the canoes and gear were on shore, the pilot brought out the map and pointed out to us our exact location, a small bay at the end of the lake. "Just around the point," he said, "you'll be at the outlet of the river."

I waved to the pilot as he did a low fly-by and then roared off. We loaded the canoes and eagerly headed out of the bay. Paddling around the point, we saw nothing but more lake. We floated around in confusion. What happened? There was supposed to be a good-sized river here. We paddled to shore to check the map. Did the pilot show us the right place on the map, but land on the wrong lake? Did he land on the right lake, but show

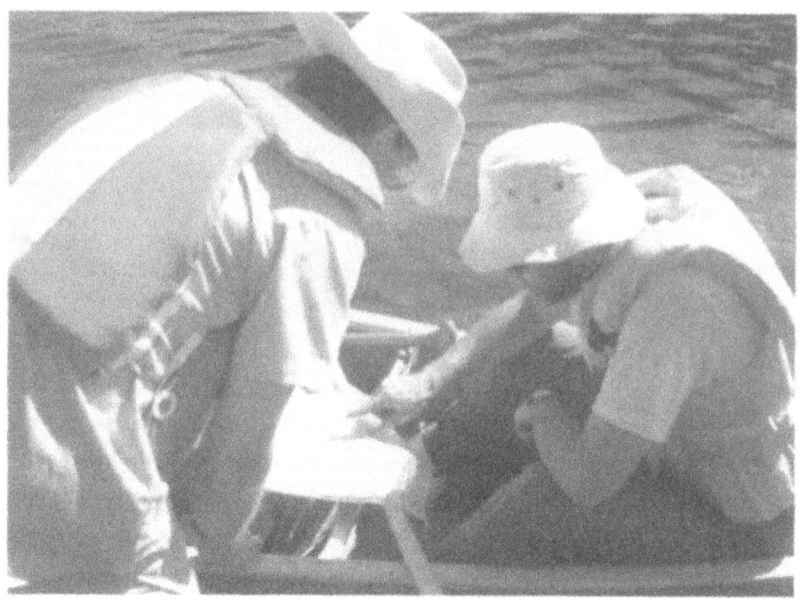
Bill and Don "bending the map" on the Foster River.

us the wrong spot on the map? We had no way of knowing.

When you travel with good maps on rivers, it's difficult to get lost. However, you have to know your starting point. So here we were on the shore of a lake somewhere in northern Saskatchewan, with no idea of our exact location. Since we had few other options, we continued to paddle down the lake. We had no real fear for ourselves, because even in northern Saskatchewan it's hard to be completely lost. As long as you head south, you will eventually hit the Churchill River.

Six kilometers later we reached the end of the lake and a river outlet. We were happy, but it didn't immediately solve our problem, as every lake in Saskatchewan ends in a river outlet: we still didn't know if this was the right one. Four or five kilometers and three rapids downriver, it became obvious that we were indeed on the right river. The pilot had put us down on the right lake, but at the wrong end. We assumed that the pilot realized his error after he took off but probably decided that since we were on the right lake we would eventually figure it out. This we did, and it turned out to be a great canoe trip. Whenever I fly in a chartered aircraft these days, I keep my eyes on the window and my finger on the map. And I make sure I know exactly where we are before I let the plane get away.

CHAPTER SIX

PEOPLE VERSUS PEOPLE

OTHING CAN RUIN A CANOE trip faster than personality conflicts within the group. When people don't get along, bad decisions are made, group support breaks down, coordination is lost, and dangerous situations can develop. The stories here are almost extreme examples of the problems that develop in such cases.

Personality problems often surface quickly on professionally guided expeditions because of the wide range of personalities inevitably represented in any group of strangers. The social expertise of canoe guides to unite total strangers into a functioning group also varies widely. Such problems are usually less severe, or at least less obvious, when friends and relatives travel together, but conflicts can still develop.

Democracy is usually the first thing to go when problems emerge; communication fails and judgment is compromised. Early recognition, preferably during pretrip planning, is key to heading off discord. Every member of the party should know the skills, goals, and motivations of the rest of the group. The decision-making process must be clear, with everyone involved. If a personality conflict or serious difference of opinion arises, the group leader should deal with it immediately. Ignoring it in the hope it will go away can lead to a breakdown in teamwork and safety awareness.

THE TRIP FROM HELL

George Drought

IGH ON THE NORTH SHORE of Lake Superior, between Wawa and Marathon, lies one of the most remote parks in Ontario, Pukaskwa National Park, and in the park is a small turbulent river called the Pukaskwa. It does not have the historical significance of rivers like the Ottawa or Missinaibi, but it is a superb wilderness river—rugged, wild, beautiful, and extremely difficult to access.

I guided a number of trips down the Pukaskwa in the early 1990s, and they were always tough seven-day trips no matter what the water level. My worst trip was in 1993, which was also my last year guiding on the river. We had three canoes. I was paddling with a client, Larry, who had told me before the trip that he lacked whitewater experience but did have some canoeing experience. In the second boat were Cathy and Ben, whom I knew to be highly experienced whitewater canoeists. My assistant guide, Pascale, was paired with a young trainee, Shelley, who would be taking Pascale's place the coming summer. Pascale was a strong paddler, and Shelley a quick study.

We met in White River on an evening in May and the next morning flew into Beaver Lake near the headwaters of the Pukaskwa. By noon, we had a camp set up on the lake, and I was putting Larry through a crash course as my bowman while Pascale did the same with Shelley. Cathy and Ben relaxed and read, but I knew that they would be fine.

I quickly realized that Larry was going to be a problem: he obviously had no canoeing experience at all, despite what he had told me. By the end of the day, I decided that we could probably do the trip in relative safety as long as he listened carefully to me. Shelley and Pascale were working well together.

We set out the next morning, and though the first couple of days were tough, there were no incidents until we reached the hydro lines just outside the borders of the park. The rapid below the hydro line is quite technical. As lead canoe, Larry and I started into it. We were about a third of the way down when I called to Larry, "Draw right!" No response.

I called again a little louder. Still no response.

Then I yelled, "Draw right!"

"Don't yell at me, you panic me!"—and then we wrapped the canoe.

The wrap was a bad one, and with the high water conditions it took me about two hours to extract the canoe. The rest of the day was uneventful, and we paddled down easy water to the Flatrock campsite, albeit with one badly creased canoe.

The next day should have been easy, as the high water had made the swifts marvelous running. The problem started when Cathy and Ben, both powerful paddlers, would not slow down and stay with the group. Our destination was Lafleur's Dam, but about four kilometers above the dam the river splits into two channels, with little apparent current at that point to indicate which way to go. We reached the fork, but there was no sign of Cathy and Ben. Which way had they gone?

I was in a quandary. I knew the correct route, but did they? Should I split up the rest of the group to go looking? Not a good idea. We waited an hour and then paddled to Lafleur's Dam to set up camp. They weren't there, either. After about two more hours, I was preparing to paddle upstream and down the other fork when they appeared, very miffed that I had not warned them about the fork.

What to say? Should I have pointed out the error they made by not waiting for us or that the high water had made the left fork look feasible, whereas in lower water the choice would have been obvious? I decided not to argue with them or embarrass them in front of the others. I hoped, however, that they had learned their lesson and would stay with us for the rest of the trip.

The paddle to our next campsite at Oxford Ledge was uneventful. But then came the days that would ruin the trip. We had to negotiate bigger, more technical rapids as the terrain dropped toward Lake Superior, and just below Oxford Ledge we entered Pukaskwa Rapids, a series of rapids and falls covering about three kilometers. The third rapid was a short, steep drop with big waves and an area where a back ferry to the right would be necessary.

I knew the rapid well and explained to everyone how it should be run. Larry and I came through safely, and Pascale and Shelley also made a clean run. Then we sat in the two canoes waiting for Cathy and Ben. For all their whitewater experience, they didn't really know how to back ferry, and they had attacked the rapid aggressively, hopping from eddy to eddy. When they finished, they berated me for not scouting the rapid and for not even considering portaging it. I pointed out that on a trip such as this—where I knew the rapids well, the canoes were fully loaded, and we didn't have sprayskirts on—strong, well-executed back paddling and ferries were mandatory skills. We paddled on to Fun Falls, a drop that can be run in medium or low water, but we all agreed to portage around due to the high water.

The next rapid brought another altercation and near disaster. The rapid cannot be run in high water, but to save themselves some carrying, Cathy and Ben elected to line the top section. Although I have reservations about lining canoes in wilderness areas, I agreed to their plan because their lining skills were good. Ben then talked Pascale and Shelley into lining as well, which I advised against. Ben put more pressure on them, and soon they started to line. Trouble began almost immediately. They let the stern out a little too far into the current, and instead of alleviating the problem by releasing the bow rope and tightening the stern, they did the opposite, dumping the canoe.

We were able to retrieve everything except one of the blue food barrels, which sped away down the rapid. Fortunately, I always carry my canoe down a portage before my packs, so it was ready to go at the bottom of the rapid. I ran the two hundred meters to the boat, jumped in, and paddled to catch the barrel, which was now bobbing through a stretch of flatwater toward the next rapid. I caught it, took it to the start of the next portage, and paddled back.

It had been too close a call, and I was not happy about what had happened. Pascale and Shelley apologized and agreed that they would listen to my advice in the future. Cathy and Ben said nothing.

The conversation at camp that night was muted, and the mosquitoes were atrocious. In the class 2 rapid right after the campsite, Larry pulled another "don't panic me!" and dumped us. I was able to swim the canoe to shore, but we were both wet and cold, and the weather was turning nasty. We decided not to change clothes, as Ringham's Gorge was just ahead. I hadn't decided whether we would attempt to run it or do the three-kilometer Two Pants Portage, an old, scarcely visible tote road on the right side of the gorge.

I decided we would paddle to the seven- or eight-meter falls at the start of the gorge, which has a tricky mountain-goat carryover on river left. I took one look at the gorge, however, and knew Larry would not be able to make it down. It was doubtful whether Pascale and Shelley could, either.

The gorge can be run by good paddlers in medium and low water, but in high water portaging is usually the safest choice. The whole gorge isn't class 5, but the location of some of the lower falls—and the force of water approaching these falls—make for risky, tight eddying.

I decided we would have to retreat upstream to the start of Two Pants Portage. The current was too strong to paddle against, so we had to wade and drag the canoes upstream the half kilometer to the start of the portage, much of the time in waist-deep water.

Ben revolted. "George, I didn't come on this river to do portages," he said. "You've said that you've been down the gorge before, so Cathy and I are going to run it."

I strongly advised Ben against it, noting that the water was higher than I had ever seen it. The argument continued, and by this time Cathy was in tears. Ben didn't care, though, he was going come hell or high water—literally.

Standing waist deep in the water I called everyone over to explain the situation and then said, "Ben, I have warned you about the dangers of Ringham's Gorge. I want you to agree in front of everyone here that you have no claim against me in the event that something goes wrong in the gorge. Furthermore, if any of my equipment, canoes, paddles, barrels, etc., should be lost or damaged, you will reimburse me. Is that clear?"

"Yes!" he replied.

"Larry, Pascale, Shelley—do you all witness this agreement between Ben and me?"

Everyone agreed. With that Cathy, still in tears, and Ben climbed into their canoe and headed downstream.

The portage was terrible. I already knew it was going to be difficult, but then the rain started. Pascale was amazing, running with canoes and packs. Shelley was more my speed and just kept plugging away. Larry was useless and became worried that we were lost, despite the fact that I had been on the portage before and knew the route. Pascale with her wilderness skills was also able to identify the route. It took us eight hours to finish the portage. We were exhausted, soaked, and covered in mud to our knees. To top it off, I slipped and wrenched my right knee (the same one I'd torn ligaments in as a youngster) on the last descent to the put-in.

The light was fading as we loaded the canoes and started paddling to the previously arranged camping spot. It was dark when we arrived, but Ben and Cathy, who had already set up their tent, did not come out to help. Pascale started a fire while Shelley and I set up the tents—including Larry's, as he just wimped out. The four of us were shivering violently, on the verge of hypothermia. Pascale prepared some hot food, and within half an hour we were well fed and warming up. Ben and Cathy refused food and still didn't emerge from their tent.

The following day the weather improved, but conversation was muted as we paddled the remaining twelve kilometers to the coast to wait for our pickup. I noticed while loading the canoes that Ben and Cathy no longer had the deck chairs that had been with them throughout the trip. Nothing was said, though, and none of the rest of us ever found out what it was like to solo down Ringham's Gorge in high water.

EDITOR: *Thorough planning allows you to develop resources and plans for nearly every eventuality, but the reactions of people in specific situations usually remain a wild card. When personalities don't mesh and trip members refuse to follow the plan during stressful, dangerous situations, chaos is the inevitable result.*

DECISIONS ON THE ARCTIC RIVER
Ric Driediger

E RECEIVED A FAX in early July from a client in Europe, "Adam." He had booked a wilderness trip with us nearly every alternate year since 1988 and was now in his early seventies. A wealthy businessman, Adam always requested a canoe trip on an Arctic river that flows into Hudson Bay alone with one guide—and always in late August.

This year, his regular guide, Kevin, was instead leading a group on the Seal River at that time. I tried to talk Adam into joining this group, but he wouldn't hear of it. Not wanting to lose his business, and looking for a way to paddle an Arctic river without paying for it on my own, I proposed to Adam by fax that I guide the trip, and he agreed.

Kevin warned me that the weather is unpredictable in the eastern Arctic by late August, and that Adam was a bit eccentric and that English was not his first language. Bad weather wasn't something that scared me: we could just sit tight, go hiking instead of canoeing, or just relax in the tent, talk, and read. I also thought I knew Adam well enough to handle his eccentricities. I wanted to discuss these things further with Kevin, but he was guiding nearly all the time, and we never really had the opportunity.

Numerous faxes and e-mails were exchanged between Europe and northern Saskatchewan before Adam and I finally agreed on a section of the Arctic River that flows between two lakes in southern Nunavut. I had never been to this area before, but after

I discussed it with others who had, it seemed like a good choice. We would fly in to a location downstream from the first lake with our intended pickup point just upstream of the second lake. We had eight days to paddle this distance—plenty of time. I had arranged with the air charter company that if we weren't at the pickup point, they would fly upriver until they found us.

We brought a personal emergency locator beacon, which if activated would alert the authorities in La Ronge who had my itinerary. They would then contact the air company to arrange emergency pickup. I also had a ground-to-air radio for contacting aircraft in the air and a shotgun for protection from bears.

We landed on the Arctic River late on August 20. After setting up the tent, Adam did something I thought strange: he made a fence of rope around the tent and hung bells from the rope in various places. He explained this was a bear fence to warn us of bear attacks during the night. In the wind, the bells rang nearly continuously. I made dinner, which, among other things, consisted of fresh meat. Adam was quite worried that this would attract bears.

We headed out the next day. Adam was quite excited by the number of caribou we saw. We stopped several times during the day to hike up onto high ridges along the river for a better view. We saw more caribou. Adam told me that to scare away the bears while we were walking we needed to continually bark like dogs. He said he had learned this method from an old trapper in a bar in Alaska. As a result, Adam was constantly barking. There was a surprising number of blueberries in the area, and I tried to explain to him that bears would be more interested in eating berries than in bothering us.

The following day we came to three waterfalls in a row that we would have to portage. Between the second and third falls, we came across dozens of dead caribou rotting along the shore. We camped below the third waterfall that night, and I made a fancy pasta meal. However, Adam refused to eat it because I had made it with river water, which he feared contained disease from the rotting caribou. Although I had boiled all the water we used, Adam wouldn't eat the pasta that night or drink any water the next day. By the end of the day, however, Adam said that if I boiled the water for ten minutes he would drink it.

The third day was beautiful. By noon, the wind had died completely for the first time on the trip, and we had almost continuously easy class 2 rapids kilometer after kilometer. The scenery was awesome. I didn't want to stop paddling, but by 5:30 p.m. we found a good place to camp shortly after the river turns north toward the second lake. The evening continued to be pleasant, and we shared a relaxing meal.

Toward morning of the fourth day I was awakened by a howling wind. It sounded like a freight train was driving over our tent. My first thought was for my canoe. The night before I had tied it loosely to a rock but had not filled it with rocks as an extra precaution. I bolted from the tent and ran down to the river. The canoe was gone! I could see marks on the gravel beach where the wind had pulled it loose from the twenty-five-kilogram rock

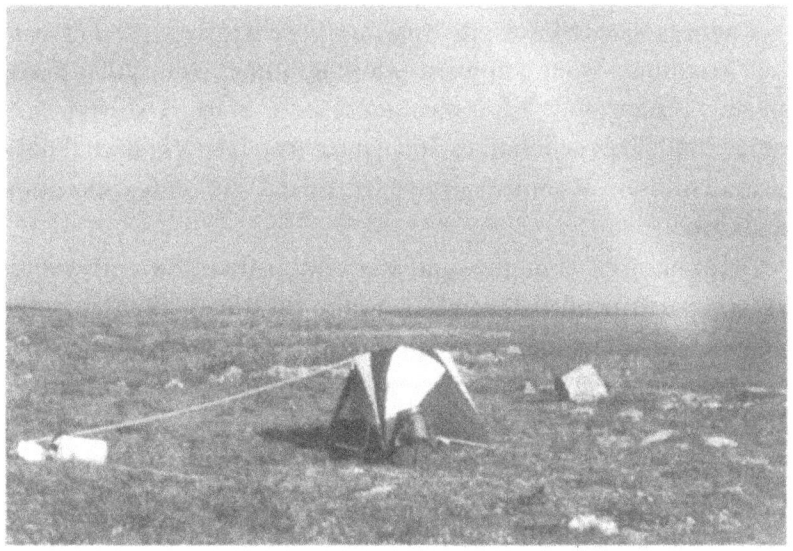

Our campsite that night on the Arctic River.

to which I had tied it. I ran several hundred meters along the shore to see if the canoe had become wedged in the rocks, then I went to inform Adam of our new situation. We both searched the riverbank, but the wind was howling from the north, with rain driving almost horizontally. The temperature was barely above freezing. After about thirty minutes Adam returned to the tent to warm up. I kept looking, even though I held little hope of finding my canoe. Soon I too retired to the tent.

I slid into my sleeping bag to stave off the chill and let my body heat warm me up.

"Did you turn on your beacon?" Adam asked.

"No," I said. "There's no emergency. The floatplane will come for us in four days."

"Oh," Adam said. "We are in a very serious situation here. Now that we can't move, the bears will find us. You have children, I have grandchildren. We must survive for them."

"Adam," I said. "We have seen no bears in four days of paddling or even any evidence of bears. When the wind dies down we can spend these days hiking and exploring. We still have a great opportunity to get to know this area, and the floatplane will find us."

"Yesterday, when you were cooking dinner, you spilled some pasta," Adam said. "You must go clean that up. The bears will smell that. They will find us and eat us. You have children, I have grandchildren. We must survive for them." Adam was pale and shaking.

I put on my wet clothes and went out. I found several strands of spaghetti from the previous night and threw them into the river, while still scanning the banks and water for a red canoe. Returning to the tent, I again tried to find some warmth in my sleeping bag. Adam asked again about the beacon.

"Adam," I explained. "Once I turn it on, I have no control over how the rescue plays out. It could cost us a small fortune. If one of us were dying, I would turn it on. Otherwise, the floatplane will find us here in four days."

"Yesterday, when you washed our dinner dishes in the river, you dropped some sauce on the bank," Adam replied. "The bears will smell that sauce and come and eat us. I have grandchildren and you have children; we must stay alive for these people. You must go clean that up."

Adam was now shaking more than before. Was it cold or panic? I went out into the cold wet wind again, found the sauce Adam was referring to, and washed it into the river. When I returned to the tent, Adam asked a third time if I had turned on the beacon. Again I replied that I hadn't.

I tried to explain to him that this system was set up for real emergencies where lives were at risk. It was difficult to know if he understood, as English was his fifth language. He asked if I was worried about the money involved. I told him that was only part of the issue. The situation simply didn't constitute an emergency; to activate the beacon would be abusing the system. He said that he would gladly pay for the rescue.

He started in again with talk of bears. "These past days you have been cooking next to the plastic barrels. I am afraid the bears will smell the food on these barrels. This will attract them, then they will eat us. You must, for our protection, wash these barrels with soap."

"Adam," I said. "It's raining hard, and the barrels *are* being washed."

"We must do this to survive. It is very important that we be around for my grandchildren and your children. You must go do this!"

I had had enough. I decided a warm sleeping bag was not worth being in the tent with Adam. Against my better judgment, I also decided to turn on my beacon, fearing that Adam's panic would only worsen. I turned it on at 8 a.m. Now it was just a matter of waiting to see what would happen.

I donned all my warm clothes and went out, running back and forth along the riverbank to warm up. Taking shelter from the elements behind a boulder, I made breakfast and coffee. Adam eventually joined me. All we could do was wait.

After breakfast, Adam went back to the tent. Minutes later he was out again—he had heard a plane! Skeptical, I sat down behind a boulder so the wind wasn't roaring in my ears. And, to my surprise, I also thought I could faintly hear a plane; then it was gone. Fifteen minutes later we heard it again. I thought it was much too early for a rescue plane to be searching for us. It seemed to be circling to the north of us. Was it looking for us? I tried the radio but couldn't raise anyone.

We couldn't hear it . . . then we could again . . . always too faint to be sure. With the wind howling in our ears it was hard to hear anything else. It was maddening. Were we hearing things? Why did it always sound the same distance away? Why was it circling? After about two hours of strained listening, I decided to ignore it.

Then, at about 11:30, I did hear something. At first I ignored it—another phantom, I decided. But moments later there was no doubt. It was a helicopter. I saw it hovering about two kilometers away, across the river and downstream. "They found my canoe," I thought. I tried the radio again and this time was successful. They flew over and landed next to our tent.

Meanwhile, another drama was playing out elsewhere. At 8:10 a.m. my wife, Theresa, had received a phone call from the La Ronge Royal Canadian Mounted Police; my beacon had been turned on. They asked if I was the kind of person who would turn it on in other than a dire emergency. She confirmed I wouldn't turn it on unless I definitely needed a rescue.

The La Ronge RCMP contacted the air charter company to rescue us, but they were experiencing winds over eighty kilometers per hour and couldn't take off. They also explained that they were unequipped to help in a medical emergency.

One after another charter company was contacted, but either high winds or mechanical difficulties made them unable to help. The La Ronge RCMP finally reached one in Rankin Inlet with a helicopter that could be ready to fly in moments. The Rankin Inlet RCMP then contacted Theresa to let her know they were airborne.

When the helicopter landed, I informed the pilot that we were OK, although I thought Adam might be suffering from mild hypothermia. The crew told us they had seen our swamped canoe stuck on a rock downstream. We packed and prepared to evacuate our gear, only to find out the chopper wouldn't have room for any of it. I was able to convince them to squeeze most of Adam's gear in and let me bring a few of my things in a daypack. We left the rest of the gear along the river.

We were wedged in so tight in the chopper that I was unable to move at all on the three-hour flight. About halfway through the nightmarish flight I woke up from an exhausted sleep to find one of the crew throwing up all over himself, and me. After what seemed like an eternity, we finally arrived in Rankin Inlet, where we were met by an emergency transport. It had been so hot in the helicopter that my concern over Adam's hypothermia was gone, so we declined medical attention.

Instead, we were driven to the local hotel and checked in. I called Theresa to reassure her that I was safe, then called the local travel agent to arrange to fly back to Saskatoon on the first flight out—three days later. Finally, I phoned the RCMP in charge of the rescue to thank him for the work he did and for keeping my wife informed throughout the procedure.

Adam and I had a good time wandering around Rankin Inlet, his earlier panic not even a memory.

When we arrived in Saskatoon, I worked out the total cost of the rescue—the cost of the equipment, hotel and meals, and flights from Rankin Inlet to Saskatoon (the helicopter flight was paid for by tax dollars).

When I presented the bill to Adam, however, he declined to pay, despite his promise on the river. Incredibly, he wanted *me* to reimburse *him* for the four days lost of the eight-day trip. We finally agreed that he would pay for the canoe trip and I would pay for the rescue. I would also give him a credit of $1,000 toward his next trip with us.

When I arrived back in Missinipe, I still had to find a way to retrieve the equipment left on the Arctic River: I had about $6,000 worth of gear sitting along the Arctic, and it would cost about $3,500 to fly up to get it. The helicopter had flown over the canoe on our way out. It was in some rapids near the shore, and I felt there was a good chance the air service could get to it. So, on the first good day, the chopper flew back to the Arctic River to get our stranded equipment.

The canoe had drifted farther downstream and out into the river. The pilot could not find most of my gear, returning with just my PFDs, two barrels of leftover food, my stove, and my camera. As far as I know, everything else is still sitting high on the bank of the Arctic River in some willows, out of sight from shore.

Not putting rocks in the canoe and then turning on the beacon cost my business about $12,000. Did I do the right thing in turning on the device? Under the circumstances, I believe so. I also believe the mistakes I made started long before we dipped a paddle in the Arctic River. I should not have gone on that trip alone with just one client. As Neil Hartling, an experienced canoe outfitter, once said, "As guides, we should not be looking for adventure—leave that for our clients." I failed my charge by being motivated by dollars and adventure. I should have paid more attention to Kevin's assessment of Adam's "eccentricities" and pressed for more information. And, once we were on the river, I should have dealt directly with Adam's fear of bears, rather than just try to mollify him.

EDITOR: *No matter how good your pretrip planning, it's impossible to predict how people you don't know well (and sometimes ones you do know well) will react to stress and danger in the wilderness. And, once again, communication is crucial to ensure everyone has the same goals and understands the risks and consequences of decisions. You just have to make the best of a bad situation.*

WHEN THINGS GO WRONG
Hap Wilson

I'S OFTEN DIFFICULT FOR wilderness expedition organizers to screen out volatile personalities merely over the phone or via e-mail. They all *sound* normal. And you can't really ask clients on the reservation form whether they suffer from some form of dementia. But as sure as the sun rises in the east, that latent psychotic behavior will surface when you're three hundred kilometers from the nearest road. In my early years as a wilderness guide, I once booked four U.S. Marines from California on the same trip as four gays from Toronto. (There really are things you can't ask the client on the reservation form!)

After that plane leaves, you're left standing on some remote riverbank looking into the faces of total strangers, praying to whatever god will listen that they have their collective shit together. And it only takes one person to foment disaster.

The single most important thing I've learned over the past thirty years as a wilderness guide is to read personalities. If you can't do this, or learn to do this early in your career, then you get out of the business quick, because if you don't you'll soon hate the job and develop a jaundiced view of the outdoor trade . . . or die from misadventure. Guiding is ten percent physical skill and ninety percent psychoanalytical ability. The only difference between a guide and a qualified analyst is the paycheck.

"You have a simple choice to make," I informed one client two days into a two-week river expedition. "Either start listening to me when I tell you not to run something, or I'll leave you here and you can walk out!" He was a lawyer, and I could tell from his expression that I was going to be next on the list of people he was suing. He still didn't listen, and the rest of us soon tired of pulling him and his canoe out of every rapid.

After a week and a half we had had enough. Against my advice he ran a class 4 chute—the same rapid that would kill a French guide the following year—and, as expected, he capsized. I paddled out to collect the canoe and gear, but left the lawyer circling in a large eddy at the base of the falls. The rest of our group ate lunch while the lawyer bobbed in and out of the whirlpool, unable to get out. He was safe enough; he just couldn't extricate himself from the current.

We rescued him a half hour later. I told him that he was welcome to sue me: I didn't own much, anyway, and I was pretty sure the six others on the trip would corroborate my side of events. We still had to deal with his sulking for four more days, but at least he didn't have the nerve to counter my call at the next rapids. Peace at a small price.

On another trip, my assistant-cum-psychopath and I were guiding two neophytes back from a trip on the Seal River. We were sailing two canoes at night down the coast of Hudson Bay to Churchill, Manitoba. My demented assistant argued for us to cross the treacherous open expanse of Button Bay to head directly for the lights of Churchill, some twenty-five kilometers away. The rest of us endorsed the safe route along the shore, and we got underway with that agreement. When it was my assistant's turn to steer, he altered course while the rest of us slept, heading out into the bay and into progressively rougher water. When we awoke and tried to regain control of the canoes, he rebelled: he was going to kill us all. This was something out of a movie thriller, except that it was actually happening—*a thwarted mutiny*. Not until I pulled out the twelve-gauge shotgun I keep tucked under the canoe spraydeck did he back off.

"It's your ship!" he announced as he tossed his paddle down to clatter on the gunwales. If he hadn't dropped his paddle, what would I have done? *Shot him?*

Then there were the thirty-two-year-old twin sisters. It was a group booking—that is, everyone knew each other. But one of the twins, a last-minute add-on to the party, had allegedly locked herself in her room for the past year, lamenting the loss of a lover who coincidentally was the best friend of the guy making the travel arrangements for the group. I was already in the bush waiting for the group to meet me at the starting point when they arrived at the floatplane base. The report that reached me, however, was that the twins, after smoking a couple of joints and removing most of their clothes, began to fondle themselves and make provocative gestures on the strut of the aircraft. At a northern air base that deals primarily with skids of cased beer and desiccated wildlife, this was quite a treat for the young pilots.

I knew there was going to be trouble as soon as I walked up to meet the plane at the put-in. The twins danced out of the plane, pirouetted off the float, shot me a "screw-you" look, and proceeded to roll around in a nearby mudhole. "That's cool," I thought, maybe it will keep the blackflies from biting.

Although even that early in my career I had learned to withstand much in the way of abuse, I did not yet feel qualified to deal with tirades. The twins refused to wear clothing, let alone shoes, which made portaging arduous and slow.

I returned to the campsite one evening to find that they had propped up over fifty lighted candles among the tinder-dry spruce. I quickly snuffed them out in deference to the fire ban. The twins hurled obscenities and death threats at me, but I stood firm.

Unbelievably, things got worse. The wife of the fellow who booked the whitewater skills course claimed that I was her soul mate. After the trip, she called my wife to demand that she divorce me so she and I could paddle off into the sunset. She then offered *her* husband to my wife in exchange.

The moral of these stories, if there is one, is that group leaders and guides should carefully evaluate all participants who sign up for a wilderness trip. Allowing one person to act as booking agent or to vouch for friends and family members is just begging for trouble. Enough mishaps occur naturally on a wilderness expedition; there's no reason to add needless personality conflicts to the mix if you can help it.

EDITOR: *While extreme, these stories demonstrate what can happen when people don't get along in the bush. Private groups aren't immune to these conflicts, either, and in some cases dealing with disagreements between friends and relatives is more difficult than with strangers. Your pretrip planning should take into account the attitudes and objectives of every member of the group.*

CHAPTER SEVEN

SOLO ADVENTURES

HERE ARE TWO KINDS of solo paddling: the first refers to one person paddling in a canoe. Then there is the kind that comes up in any discussion of canoe safety: paddling with just one canoe, regardless of the number of people in it. Paddling with one canoe has many attractions: fewer people to make mistakes; no worries about what any other canoe is doing; traveling according to your own schedule; no group decisions. However, when you have only one canoe you significantly decrease the pool of people available to point out when you're doing something stupid, to share resources, to share work, or, for that matter, to blame when things go wrong. With only one canoe, the risks are enormous, and the slightest mistake can have disastrous consequences. Anyone who chooses to paddle with only one canoe must always be aware of this risk. Every decision and action must be carefully evaluated because there is no backup; options and resources will be very limited.

GORDON RIVER BREEZES

Roger Parsons

T HE GORDON RIVER STARTS HIGH in the barrens. Flowing north and west through a series of lakes, it finally empties into the Arctic Ocean in Bathurst Inlet. Because we could find no record of anyone traveling down the Gordon, we thought a trip here would be quite an adventure. Don and I arrived at the headwaters lake at the beginning of July. We were told that ice-out had happened about two weeks earlier.

On the third day out, we portaged a long rapid that led to a lake about a kilometer wide. Our preference would have been to camp on the lakeshore at the end of the rapid, but there were fresh grizzly tracks all along the shore. To feel a little more secure, we paddled out to a small island in the middle of the lake, where we set up camp. The fishing around the island was excellent, and we had a good night's sleep.

Up early the next morning, we had breakfast and then began to break camp. I put the canoe partway into the water on a sloping rock ledge, and loaded the two canoe packs, fishing equipment, and my daypack. I was wearing a heavy green work shirt and pants, running shoes, a hat, and my PFD. I slid the boat into the water and held it, waiting for Don to join me. As he was still packing, I eased the side of the canoe onto the sloping rock and walked the fifty meters back to camp to see how he was doing. Just I reached him I felt a slight breeze and instinctively looked back at the canoe. It was already floating forty meters from shore, gliding along the surface under the gentle pressure of the breeze. I raced back to the water, threw my hat and sunglasses on the ground, and dove in.

The water was freezing, but I was in good shape and swam hard. I was just approaching the canoe, now a good hundred meters from shore, when the wind pushed it out of reach again. Twice more I chased it down, with the same result. I made up my mind that if I couldn't secure the canoe, I would keep on swimming with a steady crawl stroke, hoping to reach the mainland. On the fourth attempt, I kicked hard as I reached out, finally managing to grab the gunwale. I towed the canoe 150 meters back to the island.

Our food, clothes, tent, and other gear were in that canoe. Without quick intervention, it would have ended up on the shore of the lake some eight hundred meters away. We wouldn't have been found for at least two weeks, trapped on the small island with virtually no supplies or equipment.

It was a good lesson. The mild weather had made me careless, and we almost paid dearly.

EDITOR: *When you are paddling with only one canoe and things start to go wrong, it is a short, slippery slope to disaster.*

MIRACLE AT STANLEY MISSION
Jack Stefanyk

HE WEEKEND HAD BEEN FANTASTIC. Nine of us, mostly
teachers conducting outdoor education programs in northern Saskatchewan schools, had just completed the Basic Whitewater course with an outfitter in Missinipe, Saskatchewan. Most
of us were already fairly experienced canoeists, but the clinic
had reinforced what we knew and given us some new techniques
to work on. It was the long May weekend, and even though summer was near, winter had not relinquished its icy grip on the far
north. The Churchill was still frozen except in the vicinity of
fast-moving water and rapids.

My colleague Stan and I decided we would stop in at Little
Stanley Rapids on our way to the town of Big River. We were
coleaders in the outdoor education program at the high school
and wanted to scout the rapids for a possible school outing the
following September. Little Stanley is a small set of class 1 rapids
about three miles downriver from Stanley Mission, an isolated
native community in northern Saskatchewan.

We found that part of the river clear of ice, so we paddled our
seventeen-foot Mad River canoe from Stanley Mission to an island campsite on the south side of the rapids. We wolfed down a
hastily cooked supper, as we were anxious to get on the water to
practice the new techniques we had picked up over the weekend.
Having just completed a fairly technical clinic in rapids much
more difficult than Little Stanley, I was feeling a little cocky. As a

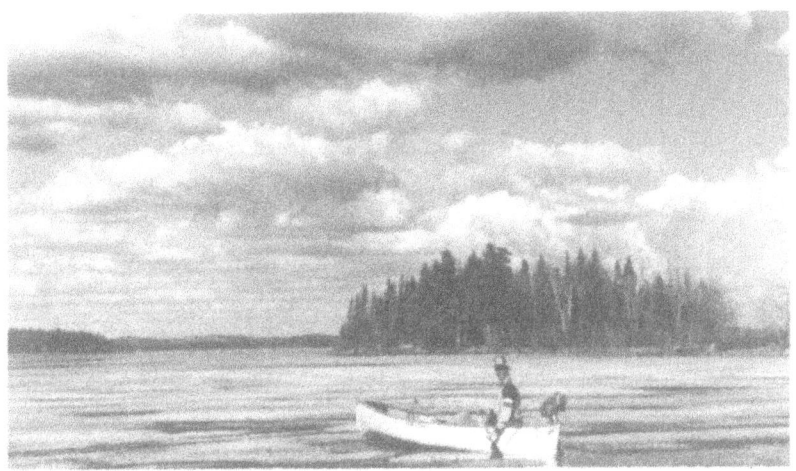

On the Churchill, headed toward the island Jack and Stan camped on.

result, we set out to "play" in this little set of rapids without wet suits, wool clothing, or the survival pouches we normally wrapped around our waists.

Little Stanley is not a long or difficult set of rapids. It starts with a little chute into some standing waves and then into fast-moving water that is split by a large rock near the end of the run. We decided that if somehow we did dump, we could brace on that rock and swing the canoe into the calm water behind it. The rapids then spill into Drope Lake, where we could still see ice farther out where the moving water lost momentum.

We were having so much fun playing in the eddies and haystacks that we lost track of the time and temperature. The cool of the evening air went unnoticed by our sweating bodies.

Then it happened. A forward ferry, which we had done dozens of times before, somehow went wrong. As we executed our "angle, motion, tilt" from an eddy to fast water, we tilted too much and over we went. Dumping in rapids is always a little scary, but this was like nothing I'd ever experienced. My body immediately began to stiffen, and I knew that we didn't have much time to get out of the icy water.

We had the presence of mind to yell to each other about the rock. As we went by I grabbed the painter and planted my feet on the edge of the rock, trying desperately to swing the canoe in behind. It didn't work. The canoe pulled me from the rock and I was again swept downriver with Stan and the canoe toward the ice in the lake.

Abandoning the canoe, I swam blindly toward shore, my arms and legs becoming less and less responsive. It felt just like a dream where there is imminent danger but you can't seem to move. Motivated by a strong will to live, I swam, thrashed, and kicked until my feet touched the rocky bottom and I could scramble shakily up the bank. I looked up to see Stan still struggling with the canoe—and drifting farther out into the lake. I also realized I was on the wrong side of the river.

Darkness was setting in, our campsite was on the other side of the river, I had no survival gear or matches, and my friend Stan was still in the freezing water. Not a good situation.

During the weekend, Stan had introduced us to a book about canoeists and kayakers who had met their bitter end. We had appropriately nicknamed it the "death book."

All I could think of as I screamed at Stan to swim to shore was that our story was going to be told in that book.

At that moment, a boat loaded with a man and his family came around the corner of our island campsite. He immediately assessed the situation and snatched Stan from the frigid water. With the canoe in tow, he swung over to pick me up and took us back to our campsite. Our rescuer was Jim, who owned a camp at Nistowiak Falls, about six miles downstream from Stanley Rapids. He had been making a trip into Stanley Mission to get supplies for the camp when he came upon us.

Feeling very lucky to be alive, Stan and I nursed our bruised egos and dried ourselves beside the fire, swearing to always remain vigilant and careful after being given this second chance, and grateful not to have become another statistic for the "death book."

HOW TO CHRISTEN A CANOE
Jim Buckingham

ERN IS THE KIND OF PERSON who thinks nothing of refinishing a paddle with nine coats of varnish, sanding lightly but thoroughly after each coat. He likes his gear to be in perfect shape, too. A little scratch on a paddle or canoe is a major embarrassment. So he was extremely proud of his brand-new Sawyer canoe, the first one we Winnipeg paddlers had seen in those days. It was British racing green, with lines so clean it looked like it was going a hundred kilometers an hour even when drifting along. Our running joke was that when Vern brought his canoe up on a beach, his girlfriend had to leap out into knee-deep water and prostrate herself on the sand so he could haul the boat up over her to protect it from scratches.

Soon after Vern's new purchase, all our friends left on a Friday night for a weekend canoe trip. I was working in a canoe store and couldn't leave until five o'clock Saturday afternoon. Vern also had to spend Saturday in town, so we decided to take off for the Shield country Saturday evening, driving like crazy to hit the water near dark, and then paddling like hell for a couple hours to join the others at their Saturday night campsite. There were a couple portages to negotiate, but we'd been over the route a few times and had a big, handheld spotlight that threw light for about half a mile. Of course we took Vern's new Sawyer: we needed the speed. It was a lake trip, no current, no rapids—we were sure we'd be fine. And we were too, until we approached the second portage.

We found the low spot on the skyline of spruce trees that marked the portage, but it was completely dark and a steady rain was falling. The shoreline, and everything else except the sky, was coal black. I pulled the big light out and swept the beam along the shore from the bow, looking for the portage, while Vern paddled us along about forty meters out. We were paralleling the shoreline, and I had the light pointed ninety degrees to our direction of travel. I called to Vern, "We shouldn't hit anything this far out."

So naturally we immediately hit a rock—a huge one. The portion above the surface was as big as a VW bus. I didn't think we were going very fast, but Vern's smooth paddling and that sleek canoe lulled us both into thinking our speed was safe. The impact was tremendous. I heard a solid crunch as the bow slammed into the rock, and we were thrown on our faces. I still can't believe we kept the canoe upright. An injury here, followed by a dark, cold swim, would have been dangerous.

Vern was quiet as we got ourselves together and continued on—at a slower pace. The ding on the bow of that brand-new Sawyer was not pretty. You can still see the mark today, thirty years later, and it always reminds us of what overconfidence can do to you.

EDITOR: *A sense of invincibility often seeps into the subconscious of experienced paddlers, leading them into dangerous situations. In this case, their impatience also encouraged Vern and Jim to set aside the caution they would otherwise have demonstrated in the reduced visibility of rain and darkness. Going solo just exacerbates the predicament.*

TROUBLE ON THE VERMILION
Doug McKown

ONNA AND DAVE WERE looking forward to an exciting, two-day canoe trip down the Vermilion River in British Columbia. The Vermilion flows west from Storm Mountain Pass on the Continental Divide, eventually joining the Kootenay River system. They were planning to paddle from the upper reaches of the river down to Canal Flats on the Kootenay River. Donna was an experienced paddler, but Dave had little river-canoeing experience. However, neither of them had ever paddled this particular section of the river.

There is little information published on the upper Vermilion River. High in the Canadian Rockies, it is a small, fast, technical mountain river. Rocks, ledges, fast currents, canyons, downed trees, and cold water make this river particularly difficult for open canoes.

Donna and Dave found this out shortly after launching their canoe in mid-July, when the river was still swollen with snowmelt. Silt reduces visibility in the water at this time of year, and as hot summer days become more common, the water level can vary significantly over the course of several hours. It wasn't long into the trip before they were in trouble. A short distance from the put-in, they approached the entrance to a small canyon. The current sped up and narrowed, limiting their ability to maneuver. In the first section of this canyon, there is a steep, narrow drop where the river pours through a crack in a limestone ledge. Although it is impossible to tell exactly where the accident occurred, Dave and Donna probably capsized at this ledge, plunging into the freezing water.

By themselves, they couldn't get the canoe and its load to shore in the powerful current. They could only hold onto the canoe for flotation, hoping to be carried into a slower section of water. They were swept down the narrow, two-kilometer canyon, trying to keep their heads above the surface of the turbulent water.

Dave lost his grip on the canoe, becoming separated from Donna. Weak and cold, he eventually washed out of the bottom of the canyon and crawled to shore. There was no sign of Donna. Making his way up to the highway, he sent for help, then went back to the river to search for Donna. Dave could barely see into the silty water around the bottom of the canyon. He found some gear but nothing else.

Eventually, the rescue service arrived to make a thorough search. Donna was not located that evening. The next day, dogs, helicopters, the Royal Canadian Mounted Police, and Warden Service Public Safety specialists were organized to continue searching. The water level of the river had dropped somewhat overnight, which allowed the rescuers to spot something in the canyon. They determined that Donna had become pinned underwater by a half-submerged log about halfway down the canyon, but the silty waters hid her on the previous day. It took the team of rescue specialists four hours to retrieve her body.

EDITOR: *Tragedies like this should never happen. If Donna and Dave had been traveling with a second canoe, the chance of immediate rescue would have increased dramatically. Proper pretrip planning and research should reveal whether a particular river is within the capabilities of the paddlers.*

SOLO ON SUPERIOR

Jim Greenacre

SOFT BREEZE CREATES SMALL RIFFLES on the surface of the lake, gently rocking my canoe. The sky is cloudless but hazy, suffusing the air with a pleasant warmth. I stop paddling and gaze around at the rugged beauty of the shoreline and the two islands off my port bow. As I glance down to remove my camera from its box, the canoe rolls gently as a slight swell passes under. I am slightly off balance, and the canoe keeps rolling. Too late to correct it, I fall out, stunned at the smooth speed of the event.

My God! This is serious. This is no warm-water lake in Algonquin Park, but Lake Superior in northern Ontario, the largest lake in the world—and one of the coldest. I watch, immobile, as the now-empty camera box and my double-blade paddle slowly float away. My life jacket. Where is my life jacket? It was on the floor behind me when I tipped. I find it under the overturned canoe. I get one arm in, but it takes several attempts to get the other arm in and the zipper closed. Not the usual canoeist's life jacket, this one looks like a long, padded vest that fits close against my body—for better protection against hypothermia. Now what?

I search my mind for anything I can remember on how a solo canoeist can execute a self-rescue in calm but deep water far from shore. Long ago on a Wilderness Canoeing Association instruction course, I saw King Baker demonstrate how to empty most of the water from a swamped canoe by rocking it violently from side to side. I try this, but it doesn't work. Maybe I can bail it out. My bailer, a large detergent bottle, is tied to a thwart. After a dozen or so scoops and dumps, I realize it's hopeless. It will take much more time than I have left. Even if I empty the canoe, how the hell am I going to climb in without help? It is difficult enough when you have a second canoe with two people steadying the opposite gunwale. Now what?

I recall bits of Red Cross water safety advice: stay with the boat . . . climb out of the water onto the boat if at all possible . . . body heat loss is less to air than to water. But this is not a boat—it's a fifteen-foot canoe with a thirty-inch beam only in the midsection.

A small black box floating beside me draws my attention: it's my hearing aid, safely waterproofed in a recycled plastic milk bag. How in the hell did it get out of my trouser pocket? I grab the box and stuff it deep inside the pocket.

The breeze is slightly offshore, and the canoe is drifting in the direction of two fair-sized islands, the ones I was about to photograph when this whole bloody mess began. The nearest island is closer than the mainland; not much, but definitely closer. Should I stay with the canoe and hope to drift into the island? Suppose I miss it—what then? This is a big lake. No, my best chance is the mainland, where I know I can walk out to my base camp and then to my truck.

Food! The small yellow stuff sack with enough food in it for about five lunches is still trapped under the spraydeck. I wrap the thin nylon drawstring around the index finger of my left hand and start swimming with a steady, measured breaststroke. I aim for a point of land jutting out between two small bays, making slow but steady progress as I wonder how much time I have before hypothermia ends my struggle. Negative thoughts. "Think positive" is the advice usually handed out by survival experts. The story of the founding of Outward Bound flashes through my mind—the sailors who survived the sinking of a ship were the ones with experience and the will to live, while younger, fit-ter sailors often gave up and drowned before help arrived. I'm going to make it. I will survive.

Something is wrong with the finger holding my food bag. It has lost all feeling. The drawstring has tightened and cut off circulation. I tread water and try to unravel it, but it's a hopeless tangle. I pull the jackknife from my trouser pocket and cut the stuff bag loose, carefully returning the knife to my pocket before starting to swim again. A few kicks with my legs and I feel something dragging on my right leg. The knife is dangling on the end of the cord that anchors it to my belt. I shake my leg and the cord frees itself. The knife will just have to dangle there.

The swell, or maybe a surface current, is pushing me off course, so I adjust my angle. A few strokes later I get a mouthful of water, then another. I must be tiring and swimming lower in the water. I decide to swim on my back to get the full benefit of the padded collar of the life jacket. It keeps my head well above the surface, but now I can't see the shore or maintain course. The two islands, now much farther away, give me a decent point of reference, and I continue.

Again I begin to review in my head the symptoms of hypothermia. I don't feel cold, and I seem to be thinking rationally; the water must be warmer than its reputation.

My right hand touches something hard. A rock. I must be close to shore. A few more kicks and my feet strike solid ground. I've made it! I roll over and crawl ashore. I'm breathing hard, sucking in great lungfuls of air.

I try to stand, but my legs won't support me. My entire body is shaking violently. Hypothermia. I know I'm well into the second stage, although I am still thinking coherently. I need a fire, external heat to help restore body heat. I manage to remove the life jacket and the bush jacket, though I have trouble with the buttons on the bush jacket.

The beach is littered with driftwood, and I soon have a pile of kindling ready. I try to strike a match, then again, but it's no use—

I just can't stop shaking. I give up, lying back to feel the warmth of the rocks beneath me. My shirt is open to the waist, and the cold flesh soaks up life-restoring warmth from the sun.

Gradually the shivering subsides enough that I can control my hands, though my legs and feet are still slow to respond. I crawl over to the heap of kindling, this time using my lighter on a small piece of birch bark. Four flicks to get a spark, five flicks for a small flame. The birch bark catches instantly and I have a fire. Within minutes I have a bonfire, and soon I'm able to stand.

By now I am feeling rested and am thinking of food. The half loaf of rye bread is slightly damp on one corner, and the margarine is OK in a plastic jar. I reach into my trouser pocket for my jackknife—it's gone. All I have left is the length of cord, which is supposed to prevent such a thing from happening. The hearing aid has also disappeared from my trouser pocket.

After lunch, I make my way over to the point and search the water for some sign of my canoe. Something small and bright on the tip of the island catches my eye. That must be my yellow canoe, but it doesn't help me much right now.

I know precisely where I am, and the topo map tells me that about a kilometer due east is a trail leading back to Gargantua Harbour, where I'm camped. I decide it's best to stay close to the shore as much as possible. Walking is easy on the pebble beaches, but many of the points between bays rise straight out of the water, so I have to make bushwhacking detours inland. Two hours later I check my position on the map. The trail should now be close to the shoreline, so on a compass bearing I head due east. I find the trail after a hundred meters or so. Another fifteen minutes and I'm packing up my base camp and hiking the two kilometers back to my truck.

It was a day and a half before I could find someone to take me out to the island in a motorboat. A thirty-minute ride under full power brought me to the island, and there, lodged in a fissure in the rock wall, is my little yellow canoe.

How long was I in the water? Almost too long. I know where I swamped and where I crawled ashore; measuring in a straight line on the topo map, I calculate I swam somewhere between 1,000 and 1,100 meters. I had broken a cardinal rule of safe canoeing, as many of us do: never canoe alone.

EDITOR: *Sometimes when you are traveling with just one canoe and everything is going smoothly, you forget that you're actually by yourself. A simple mistake, one that would be harmless with another canoe around, can be deadly.*

CHAPTER EIGHT

IT'S ALL ABOUT SAFETY AWARENESS

N SPITE OF ALL THE MISTAKES, misjudgments, inattention, impatience, complacency, and carelessness, most canoeing disasters have happy endings, in which luck and survival skills each play a role. Hopefully, you get the chance to survive your mistakes and learn from them.

While the experiences described in these stories provide many specific lessons, pretrip planning and safety awareness remain the most valuable. You must assume that anything that can go wrong on a canoe trip eventually will. Detailed planning for a wilderness canoe trip is a complex operation, but here are guidelines to help you develop a system of your own.

Make sure you know as much as possible about all the conditions you are likely to encounter. What is the technical difficulty of the route? What extremes of weather and water conditions are possible? Are dangerous animals in the area? Where are your rescue resources and how can you contact them?

A clear understanding of the skills, experience, and objectives of all the members of the group is essential for safe traveling. The overall difficulty of the trip must correspond with the skills of the *least* experienced participants.

Having the proper equipment, in good working order, should be the easiest part of staying safe. However, the amount and type of equipment depends on the conditions you may face. Even the smallest incident can mean trouble if you don't have the proper equipment to deal with it. This can range from the right kind of canoe to proper medical supplies to emergency beacons. Think first, survive later.

Some concepts seem so simple. If you're traveling in bear country, be prepared to encounter bears. Keep a clean camp and store food properly. Deterrents such as pepper spray or firearms may be your only practical defense against determined bruins. Have deterrents with you, know how to use them, and have a plan in mind. Don't just assume you won't encounter bears.

With detailed knowledge of the route, appropriate supplies and resources, and an understanding of the strengths and weaknesses of the paddlers in your group, you can start making contingency plans for emergencies. Contingency plans should be discussed with the group before setting out so everyone has a good idea of the options and resources available if your plans need to change quickly.

Practice is a concept often ignored by paddling groups. Successful rescue techniques and paddling skills don't develop magically. Everyone should review the rescue plans as well as physically practice using the skills and equipment in a controlled situation before venturing out. Practicing common rescue scenarios gives paddlers a better understanding of basic procedures in any emergency and ensures that all resources and options are put to the best use.

One of the most important elements of pretrip planning is assessing the level of risk participants are willing to accept. The risks associated with the trip, and with all activities involved in the trip, must be clear to all participants. Risk is based on the difficulty of the trip, the potential hazards, the probability of incidents occurring, and most importantly, the severity of those incidents. The more remote the area, the fewer the resources available to deal with serious problems.

Understanding risk is critical on solo trips. Paddling with just one canoe is not necessarily a bad idea, just hazardous. Simple problems can escalate quickly into life-threatening situations. Plan carefully, and pay particular attention to equipment and how you will access resources.

The goal of pretrip planning is always to maximize your options. Comprehensive planning, good equipment, and skilled, experienced paddlers translate to more options when disaster strikes. The more limited your options are, the greater is the risk of the activity.

When your trip is actually underway, safety awareness becomes paramount. No matter how well you plan, things can still go wrong due to poor decisions or random events beyond your control. The key is to deal with a bad situation as early as possible to prevent additional complications.

To make a good decision, you first need a clear, well-defined objective and full information. Getting all the information is the tricky part. It may be as simple as thoroughly scouting a rapid before deciding whether or not to run it or as difficult as factoring in the severity of an injury, the weather and terrain, and paddling skills while planning an evacuation. If the decision being made involves the entire group, everyone has to understand the consequences of the decision. Paddlers must never hesitate to speak up if they aren't willing to take a particular risk or if they are aware of a minor problem or conflict that could escalate into serious trouble.

Remember that skills and experience are not transferable. You can't depend on your abilities to get a less skilled or less experienced paddler through a difficult situation, just as you should not depend on someone else's skills to protect you. Always be aware of the abilities of all members of the group when deciding how to deal with a potentially dangerous situation.

Poor communication is probably the biggest contributor to chaos. Anyone who has done much tandem river canoeing knows how hard it is to keep track of what the other person in your own canoe is doing or intending to do. Making sure that everyone in a group knows what's going on can be a considerable task. One of the best techniques for maintaining clear communications is to keep the group together so you can make or change plans, ask questions, and stay aware. As soon as you separate, that vital communications link is gone, and plans break down.

When you do decide on a particular plan of action, make sure that all members of the group clearly understand what is going to take place. Explain the activity in detail, go over it again, ask for questions, and once you're sure that everyone understands, go over the plan yet again.

All the pretrip planning and group decision making doesn't mean a thing unless you remain constantly alert in the field. You need to recognize instantly when something isn't quite right and take appropriate steps to rectify the problem before the situation gets out of hand. Safety awareness is more difficult than it sounds. Much of the joy in paddling lies in relaxing and enjoying the day, but this leads to complacency, inattention, and carelessness. Having everyone keep an eye on each other helps combat problems, but it eventually comes down to the individual: each person must think past the decision to understand the consequences of the action.

Whenever I make a decision, the first thing I do is *stop*. I sit for a minute or two and think through the plan. I think about all the consequences I might suffer if the plan fails. What if the weather doesn't cooperate? . . . what if that forest fire comes this way? . . . what if I capsize in freezing water? . . . what if someone gets hurt? . . . what if they don't make that ferry? . . . Once I get my mind around the risks, I can better judge if I am making the right decision. Of course, this is all much harder when you are tired, sleepy, cold, or being rained on. Simple decisions are often the most dangerous because you don't really believe that anything could go wrong.

I sometimes try to imagine what it would be like to tell my story later. Would it sound like I was doing something smart or something stupid? The best choice is often the hardest one—stopping the trip; backtracking to a long, ugly portage; lining instead of running a rapid; retracing your route. Realistic assessment of consequences and risk will always help you make a better decision.

When you are out canoeing and something—anything—happens that you don't feel comfortable with, "just say no." Stop to think before you paddle, and you'll paddle longer.

RECOMMENDED READING

Canoeing Manitoba Rivers, John Buchanan (Calgary, Alberta: Rocky Mountain Books, 1997)

Canoeing Safety and Rescue, Doug McKown (Calgary, Alberta: Rocky Mountain Books, 1992)

Expedition Canoeing: A Guide to Canoeing Wild Rivers in North America, 3rd ed., Cliff Jacobson (Guilford, Connecticut: Globe Pequot Press, 2001)

Northern Saskatchewan Canoe Trips: A Guide to Fifteen Wilderness Rivers, Laurel Archer (Erin, Ontario: Boston Mills Press, 2003)

Sea Kayaker's Deep Trouble: True Stories and Their Lessons from Sea Kayaker Magazine, Matt Broze and George Gronseth, edited by Christopher Cunningham (Camden, Maine: Ragged Mountain Press, 1997)

Whitewater Rescue Manual: New Techniques for Canoeists, Kayakers, and Rafters, Charles Walbridge and Wayne A. Sundmacher Sr. (Camden, Maine: Ragged Mountain Press, 1995)

The Wilderness Paddler's Handbook, Alan S. Kesselheim (Camden, Maine: Ragged Mountain Press, 2001)

ORGANIZATIONS

American Canoe Association
7432 Alban Station Boulevard,
Suite B-232
Springfield, Virginia 22150
703-451-0141
www.acanet.org

Canadian Recreational
Canoeing Association
P.O. Box 398
446 Main Street West
Merrickville, Ontario
K0G 1N0 CANADA
888-252-6292
www.crca.ca

Health and Safety Services
American Red Cross
2025 East Street, Northwest
Washington, D.C. 20006
202-303-4498
www.redcross.org/services/hss/
index.html

Horizons Unlimited—
Churchill River Canoe
Outfitters
Box 1110
La Ronge, Saskatchewan
S0J 1L0 CANADA
888-511-2726
www.churchillrivercanoe.com

Minnesota Canoe Association
Box 13567
Dinkytown Station
Minneapolis, Minnesota
55414
952-985-1111
www.canoe-kayak.org

Red Cross Water Safety
Services
Canadian Red Cross
170 Metcalfe Street, Suite 300
Ottawa, Ontario
K2P 2P2 CANADA
613-740-1900
www.redcross.ca/english/
watersafety/

Wilderness Canoe Association
P.O. Box 91068
2901 Bayview Avenue
Toronto, Ontario
M2K 2Y6 CANADA
http://wildernesscanoe.ca
(Canadian)
www.wildernesscanoe.org
(U.S.)

LAUREL ARCHER

Laurel Archer and Brad Koop, her paddling partner in "Meeting the Big Wheel at the Wheeler," met as canoe guides on the Churchill River in northern Saskatchewan in 1988. They have since paddled rivers from the Canadian tundra to the Grand Canyon to Costa Rica and Mongolia. After losing their log home on Lac la Ronge to a forest fire, they headed west to Vancouver Island for new adventures. They now experience the serious difficulty of deciding whether to go kayak surfing, whitewater paddling, sea kayaking, or canoe tripping in a climate that permits year-round paddling!

MEL BAUGHMAN

Mel began canoeing as a teenager and honed his outdoor skills on rivers and lakes throughout the American Midwest and southern Canada. On his many extensive canoe trips, Mel enjoys fishing and photography. Now an experienced wilderness canoeist, Mel is known for his attention to detail in trip planning and organization. He has been the editor of *Hut!*,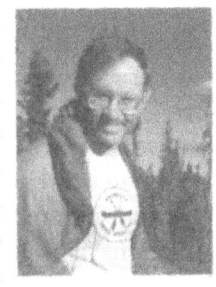
the magazine of the Minnesota Canoe Association, and organizes

GEORGE DROUGHT

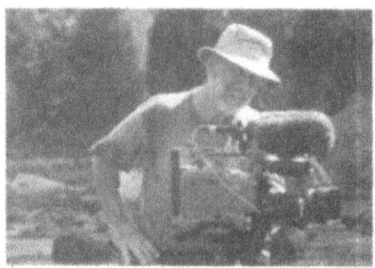

George Drought was born in England in 1938. As a teenager he was an avid hiker and outdoors enthusiast, and within two weeks of his arrival in Canada in 1956 he began his first solo canoe trip. He has accumulated years of paddling in Ontario, Québec, Manitoba, the Northwest Territories, and Nunavut. He is a qualified Ontario tripping and whitewater instructor and a founding member of the Barrie Canoe Club. George has written a number of articles about his whitewater adventures, as well as guides to the Petawawa and Madawaski rivers. Since 1986 he and his wife, Barbara, have run a wilderness tripping company, to which they've added a video production company. They spend most of their time doing what they like best—partaking in, and introducing others to, the joys of whitewater paddling through film and the written word.

JIM GREENACRE

Jim Greenacre emigrated from England to Canada in 1952, settled in Toronto, and has made his home there ever since. He was introduced to paddling on a week-long canoe trip in Algonquin Provincial Park in 1975, and 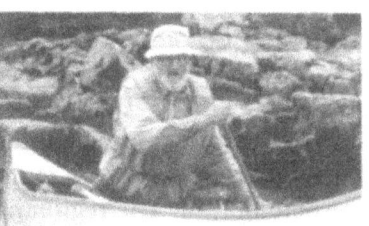 never looked back. An avid outdoorsman, Jim has paddled among the Queen Charlotte Islands, along the shores of Labrador, across the Arctic, and on many rivers and lakes between.

DEAN GYUG

Dean began canoeing at age thirteen, and there followed many family trips in Saskatchewan and Alberta, including the little disaster on northern Saskatchewan's Clearwater River that he chronicles here. At sixteen Dean took up kayaking and has made numerous trips all across western Canada. Like many paddlers, his favorite paddling area is the wild shield country of northern Saskatchewan and Manitoba, a land of awesome rapids, perfect solitude, and great fishing.

TONI HARTING

Toni Harting is a freelance writer-photographer specializing in canoe-related nature subjects. He is the editor of *Nastawgan*, the quarterly journal of the Wilderness Canoe Association, and has published two books on canoeing: *French River: Canoeing the River of Sticks* and *Shooting Paddlers: Photographic Adventures with Canoeists, Kayakers and Rafters*. Toni makes his home in Toronto.

BOB HENDERSON AND WARREN TRIMBLE

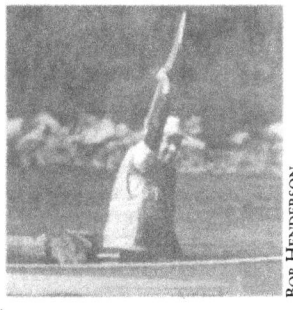

Bob Henderson teaches Outdoor Education at McMaster University, Hamilton, Ontario. Bob has extensive canoeing experience and is a regular contributor for *Kanawa: Canada's Canoeing and Kayaking Magazine*.

Warren Trimble (see photo), a teacher in Hamilton, Ontario, splits his year between Hamilton and the Edmonton-Jasper area, paddling watersheds east and west.

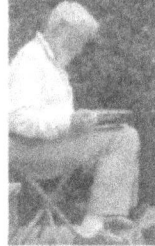

BILL HOSFORD

Bill Hosford is a professor of materials science and engineering at the University of Michigan and has been canoeing in Canada almost every summer since 1964. He has paddled the Missinaibi, Pukaskwa, East Pukaskwa, Steel, Batchewana, Sand, Magpie, Winisk, and Severn rivers in Ontario; the Rupert in Québec; the Nahanni, Mountain, Horton, and Coppermine in the Northwest Territories; and the Thelon and Burnside in Nunavut. He prefers groups of two or three canoes, traveling light, but he packs watercolors and tries to paint at least one picture per day.

CLIFF JACOBSON

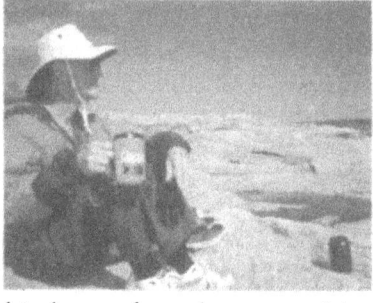

Cliff Jacobson is a professional canoe guide for the Science Museum of Minnesota, a wilderness canoeing consultant, and the author of more than a dozen books on camping and canoeing. He recently retired from teaching middle school environmental science and plans to split his time among canoeing, camping, and sharing his love of outdoor travel by writing and teaching about it. When he is not writing, speaking, or leading canoe trips in Canada, he is out paddling his solo canoe or figuring out a new way to improve his equipment.

JOHN LENTZ

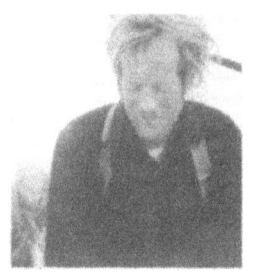

John Lentz has been paddling wilderness rivers since 1962, when he was part of the third party to descend the length of the Back—after George Back in 1834 and HBC Chief Factor James Anderson in 1855. Since then, John has completed fourteen trips in northern Canada and two in Siberia. In 1983, at the end of Wilberforce Canyon on the Hood River, his party found artifacts left by the Franklin Expedition in 1821. John is a fellow of the Explorers Club and a member of the Royal Geographical Society. When not on a northern stream, John is a financial analyst for a Washington consulting firm.

PAM LITTLE

Pam Little grew up paddling in Manitoba and has extensive canoe-tripping experience across western and northern Canada. She makes her home in Banff, Alberta, where she works as an emergency room nurse. Pam continues to paddle recreationally and participates in wilderness canoe trips whenever she has time.

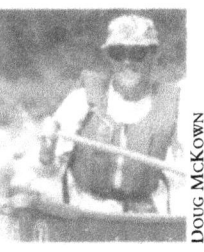

DOUG MCKOWN

DEAN MCLEOD

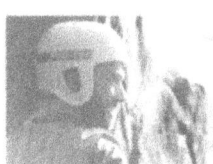

Dean McLeod grew up canoeing in Manitoba. He has extensive experience throughout western Canada, including work as a wilderness tripping guide for Enviros. In the early 1980s Dean was a river canoe instructor at the Banff National Army Cadet Camp. He and his family reside in Winnipeg, where he teaches high school.

ROGER PARSONS

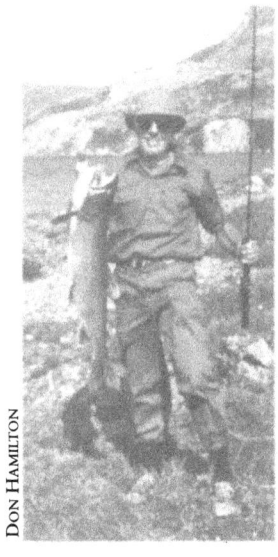

DON HAMILTON

Roger Parsons has influenced the sport of canoeing in Canada for more than forty years. He was the moving force in the development of closed-boat whitewater racing in that country and was a member of the International Canoeing Federation's Slalom and Wildwater Committee for many years. One of Roger's many lasting accomplishments was the creation of the Minden Wild Water Preserve, Canada's premiere whitewater training facility. He has paddled in many countries but has a special love for Canada's last frontier, the Arctic. Retired and living in Barrie, Ontario, Roger maintains a busy paddling schedule.

LEE PEARSON

Lee Pearson works as a lawyer and teacher in Ontario. But he's also an experienced paddler with many interesting canoe trips to his credit. Lee and his wife, Gail, have paddled many rivers in Ontario, Saskatchewan, Manitoba, and the Northwest Territories.

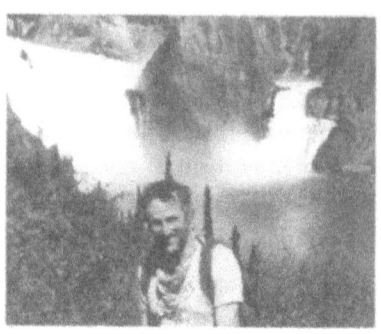

SARA SEAGER AND MIKE WEVRICK

Sara Seager and Mike Wevrick met on a Wilderness Canoe Association trip in early 1994 and have been paddling together ever since. (The canoe trip described in this book was their honeymoon.) Originally from Canada, they have been living (and paddling) in the northeast United States for the past seven years, gradually migrating south. They live in Princeton, New Jersey, where Sara is an astrophysicist and Mike a science textbook editor. They have been canoe tripping for seventeen and twenty-five years, respectively, and still manage to spend a month each summer paddling in northern Canada with their dog, Kira, who loves the wilderness as much as they do.

JOHN SILVER

John Silver makes his home in Winnipeg, where he has been an educator for the past twenty-two years. Through paddling, John has seen the rich wilderness of Canada up to the Arctic Circle, challenging himself physically and spiritually in settings where life actually makes sense at times. John's paddling experiences would not have been possible without the cooperation of his wife of twenty-seven years, Pat, and that all-important group of paddling friends, Deb, Al, Blake, and Dwight.

JACK STEFANYK

Jack Stefanyk lives in British Columbia, where he has been teaching for the past sixteen years. Decades of canoeing have taken him all over Saskatchewan, Manitoba, and the Northwest Territories. He has also worked as a canoe guide for the Nemeiben Lake Bible and Canoe Camp. When not canoeing, Jack enjoys an active life with his wife and two children.

HAP WILSON

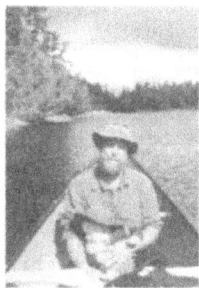 Hap Wilson is a self-taught artist, writer, photographer, and wilderness guide. His work reflects his love for the few remaining pockets of true wilderness and is inspired by the natural and supernatural worlds, which he has experienced on numerous canoe adventures throughout Canada. Hap has written and illustrated over eight books about the Canadian wilderness including *Voyages*, which won the Natural Resources Council of America award for the best environmental book of 1995. His latest book is *Canoeing and Hiking Wild Muskoka: An Eco-Adventure Guide*. Hap operates Eskakwa Wilderness Adventures and Retreat with his wife Stephanie and guides trips in Temagami, Québec, and the barrenlands.

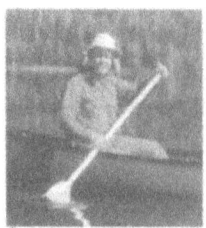

Since DOUG McKOWN began canoeing in the 1960s, he has paddled rivers all over North America. A certified canoe instructor (Alberta Recreational Canoe Association and Canadian Recreational Canoe Association) for many years, he has taught university and adult education canoeing courses and has directed many paddling programs, including a nine-year stint at Banff National Army Cadet Camp.

Doug created canoeing and river rescue programs for organizations such as Parks Canada, Continuing Education, and the Royal Canadian Department of Defense. A well-published author of articles on canoeing, he has also written *Canoeing Safety and Rescue: A Handbook of Safety and Rescue Procedures for Lake and River Canoeists*. Doug still manages to get out on the water an average of fifty days each year, despite working full-time as an advanced life support paramedic in Banff, Alberta.

DO YOU HAVE A STORY TO TELL?

I'm always interested in hearing stories about canoeing adventures and misadventures. If you have been thinking "been there, done that" while reading these stories, I'd like to hear from you. From the smallest incidents to major disasters, learning about the problems faced by other canoeists can make us all better paddlers. Send your stories to me at mckown@expertcanmore.net.

Ingram Content Group UK Ltd.
Milton Keynes UK
UKHW022025190323
418794UK00011B/266